W0259609

Cram101 Textbook Outlines to accompany:

Asthma and COPD : Basic Mechanisms and Clinical Management

Peter Barnes, 1st Edition

Learning System

Cram101 Textbook Outlines is a learning system. The notes in this book are the highlights of your textbook, you will never have to highlight a book again.

How to use this book. Take this book to class, it is your notebook for the lecture. The notes and highlights on the left hand side of the pages follow the outline and order of the textbook. All you have to do is follow along while your instructor presents the lecture. Circle the items emphasized in class and add other important information on the right side. With Cram101 Textbook Outlines you'll spend less time writing and more time listening. Learning becomes more efficient.

Cram101.com Online

Increase your studying efficiency by using Cram101.com's practice tests and online reference material. It is the perfect complement to Cram101 Textbook Outlines. Use self-teaching matching tests or simulate in-class testing with comprehensive multiple choice tests, or simply use Cram's true and false tests for quick review. Cram101.com even allows you to enter your in-class notes for an integrated studying format combining the textbook notes with your class notes.

Visit **www.Cram101.com**, click Sign Up at the top of the screen, and enter **DK73DW15737** in the promo code box on the registration screen. Your access to www.Cram101.com is discounted by 50% because you have purchased this book. Sign up and stop highlighting textbooks forever.

 ISBN(s): 9781614614500. PUBR-7.201146

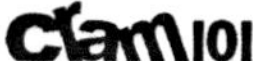

Asthma and COPD : Basic Mechanisms and Clinical Management
Peter Barnes, 1st

CONTENTS

Chapter 1. Definitions, Epidemiology, and Genetics of Asthma and COPD

Asthma	Asthma is characterized by a predisposition to chronic inflammation of the lungs in which the airways (bronchi) are reversibly narrowed. Asthma affects 7% of the population of the United States, 6.5% of British people and a total of 300 million worldwide. During Asthma attacks (exacerbations of Asthma), the smooth muscle cells in the bronchi constrict, the airways become inflamed and swollen, and breathing becomes difficult.
Disease	A disease or medical condition is an abnormal condition of an organism that impairs bodily functions, associated with specific symptoms and signs. It may be caused by external factors, such as invading organisms, or it may be caused by internal dysfunctions, such as autoimmune diseases. In human beings, \`disease\` is often used more broadly to refer to any condition that causes pain, dysfunction, distress, social problems, and/or death to the person afflicted, or similar problems for those in contact with the person.
Lung	The Lung or pulmonary system is the essential respiration organ in all air-breathing animals, including most tetrapods, a few fish and a few snails. In mammals and the more complex life forms, the two Lungs are located in the chest on either side of the heart. Their principal function is to transport oxygen from the atmosphere into the bloodstream, and to release carbon dioxide from the bloodstream into the atmosphere.
Obstructive lung disease	Obstructive lung disease is a category of respiratory disease characterized by airway obstruction. MeSH includes the following in this category: · Asthma · Bronchitis · Chronic obstructive pulmonary disease Cystic fibrosis is sometimes also included in this category. FEV1/FVC ratio is usually decreased.

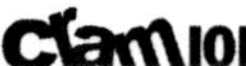

Chapter 1. Definitions, Epidemiology, and Genetics of Asthma and COPD

Protein	Proteins are organic compounds made of amino acids arranged in a linear chain and folded into a globular form. The amino acids in a polymer chain are joined together by the peptide bonds between the carboxyl and amino groups of adjacent amino acid residues. The sequence of amino acids in a protein is defined by the sequence of a gene, which is encoded in the genetic code.
Chronic obstructive pulmonary disease	Chronic obstructive pulmonary disease refers to chronic bronchitis and emphysema, a pair of two commonly co-existing diseases of the lungs in which the airways become narrowed. This leads to a limitation of the flow of air to and from the lungs causing shortness of breath. In contrast to asthma, the limitation of airflow is poorly reversible and usually gets progressively worse over time.
Inflammation	Inflammation is the complex biological response of vascular tissues to harmful stimuli, such as pathogens, damaged cells, or irritants. Inflammation is a protective attempt by the organism to remove the injurious stimuli as well as initiate the healing process for the tissue. Inflammation is not a synonym for infection.
Surfactant	Surfactants are wetting agents that lower the surface tension of a liquid, allowing easier spreading, and lower the interfacial tension between two liquids. The term Surfactant is a blend of surface active agent. Surfactants are usually organic compounds that are amphiphilic, meaning they contain both hydrophobic groups (their `tails`) and hydrophilic groups (their `heads`).
Allergen	An Allergen is a nonparasitic antigen capable of stimulating a type-I hypersensitivity reaction in atopic individuals. Most humans mount significant Immunoglobulin E responses only as a defense against parasitic infections. However, some individuals mount an IgE response against common environmental antigens.
Colitis	Colitis is a chronic digestive disease characterized by inflammation of the colon. Colitis is one of a group of conditions which are inflammatory and auto-immune, affecting the tissue that lines the gastrointestinal system (the large and small intestine). It is classed as an inflammatory bowel disease (IBD), not to be confused with irritable bowel syndrome (IBS).

Erythromycin	Erythromycin is a macrolide antibiotic that has an antimicrobial spectrum similar to or slightly wider than that of penicillin, and is often used for people who have an allergy to penicillins. For respiratory tract infections, it has better coverage of atypical organisms, including mycoplasma and Legionellosis. It was first marketed by Eli Lilly and Company, and it is today commonly known as EES (Erythromycin ethylsuccinate, an ester prodrug that is commonly administered).
Factor XII	Hageman factor is a plasma protein , an enzyme (EC 3.4.21.38) of the serine protease (or serine endopeptidase) class. In humans, Factor XII is encoded by the F12 gene. It is part of the coagulation cascade and activates factor XI and prekallikrein.
Ulcerative colitis	Ulcerative colitis (Colitis ulcerosa, Ulcerative colitis) is a form of inflammatory bowel disease (IBD). Ulcerative colitis is a form of colitis, a disease of the intestine, specifically the large intestine or colon, that includes characteristic ulcers, or open sores, in the colon. The main symptom of active disease is usually constant diarrhea mixed with blood, of gradual onset.
Usual interstitial pneumonia	Usual interstitial pneumonia, commonly abbreviated Usual interstitial pneumonia, is the name of a histopathological pattern seen in diffuse lung diseases, i.e. interstitial lung diseases. It is classified as an idiopathic interstitial pneumonia, and may be idiopathic, i.e. the cause is unknown, or due to a known cause, e.g. asbestos exposure. The hallmarks of Usual interstitial pneumonia are interstitial inflammation, i.e. inflammation of the alveolar walls, and fibrosis (scarring).
Variability	The term Variability, \`the state or characteristic of being variable\`,describes how spread out or closely clustered a set of data is. This may be applied to many different subjects: · Climate Variability · Genetic Variability · Heart rate Variability · Human Variability · Solar van · Spatial Variability

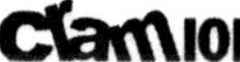

· Statistical Variability

· Variability

Volume

The Volume of any solid, liquid, gas, plasma, or vacuum is how much three-dimensional space it occupies, often quantified numerically. One-dimensional figures (such as lines) and two-dimensional shapes (such as squares) are assigned zero Volume in the three-dimensional space. Volume is commonly presented in units such as cubic meters, cubic centimeters, liters, or milliliters.

Leukocytes

White blood cells are cells of the immune system defending the body against both infectious disease and foreign materials. Five different and diverse types of Leukocytes exist, but they are all produced and derived from a multipotent cell in the bone marrow known as a hematopoietic stem cell. Leukocytes are found throughout the body, including the blood and lymphatic system.

Neuroendocrine

Neuroendocrine [IPA nÊŠÉ™roÊŠË'É›ndÉ™krÉªn] cells are cells that release a hormone into the circulating blood in response to a neural stimulus. These hormones may be amines, neuropeptides, or specialized amino acids. They package the hormones in vesicles and send these packages via long processes to blood vessels.

Connective tissue

Connective tissue is a form of fibrous tissue. It is one of the four types of tissue in traditional classifications (the others being epithelial, muscle, and nervous tissue).

Collagen is the main protein of Connective tissue in animals and the most abundant protein in mammals, making up about 25% of the total protein content.

Fiber types as follows:

· collagenous fibers

· elastic fibers

· Bone Marrow

Various Connective tissue conditions have been identified; these can be both inherited and environmental.

· Marfan syndrome - a genetic disease causing abnormal fibrillin.

· Scurvy - caused by a dietary deficiency in vitamin C, leading to abnormal collagen.

· Ehlers-Danlos syndrome - deficient type III collagen- a genetic disease causing progressive deterioration of collagens, with different EDS types affecting different sites in the body, such as joints, heart valves, organ walls, arterial walls, etc.

· Loeys-Dietz syndrome - a genetic disease related to Marfan syndrome, with an emphasis on vascular deterioration.

· Pseudoxanthoma elasticum - an autosomal recessive hereditary disease, caused by calcification and fragmentation of elastic fibres, affecting the skin, the eyes and the cardiovascular system.

· Systemic lupus erythematosus - a chronic, multisystem, inflammatory disorder of probable autoimmune etiology, occurring predominantly in young women.

· Osteogenesis imperfecta (brittle bone disease) - caused by insufficient production of good quality collagen to produce healthy, strong bones.

· Fibrodysplasia ossificans progressiva - disease of the Connective tissue, caused by a defective gene which turns Connective tissue into bone.

· Spontaneous pneumothorax - collapsed lung, believed to be related to subtle abnormalities in Connective tissue.

· Sarcoma - a neoplastic process originating within Connective tissue.

Pelvic inflammatory disease

Pelvic inflammatory disease (or disorder) is a generic term for inflammation of the female uterus, fallopian tubes, and/or ovaries as it progresses to scar formation with adhesions to nearby tissues and organs. This may lead to tissue necrosis and sometimes abscess formation whereby pus can be released into the peritoneum. Pelvic inflammatory disease is often associated with sexually transmitted infections, as it is a common result of such infections.

Growth factor	A Growth factor is a naturally occurring substance capable of stimulating cellular growth, proliferation and cellular differentiation. Usually it is a protein or a steroid hormone. Growth factors are important for regulating a variety of cellular processes.
Atherosclerosis	Atherosclerosis is a condition in which an artery wall thickens as the result of a build-up of fatty materials such as cholesterol. It is a syndrome affecting arterial blood vessels, a chronic inflammatory response in the walls of arteries, in large part due to the accumulation of macrophage white blood cells and promoted by low-density lipoproteins (plasma proteins that carry cholesterol and triglycerides) without adequate removal of fats and cholesterol from the macrophages by functional high density lipoproteins (HDL), . It is commonly referred to as a hardening or furring of the arteries.
Group B Streptococcus	Infection with Group B Streptococcus can cause serious illness and , especially in newborn infants, the elderly, and patients with compromised immune systems. Group B streptococci are also prominent veterinary pathogens, because they can cause bovine mastitis (inflammation of the udder) in dairy cows. The species name \`agalactiae\` meaning \`no milk\`, alludes to this.
Pathology	Pathology is the study and diagnosis of disease through examination of organs, tissues, bodily fluids, and whole bodies (autopsies). The term also encompasses the related scientific study of disease processes, called General Pathology. Medical Pathology is divided in two main branches, Anatomical Pathology and Clinical Pathology.
Defensins	Defensins are small cysteine-rich cationic proteins found in both vertebrates and invertebrates. They are active against bacteria, fungi and many enveloped and nonenveloped viruses. They consist of 18-45 amino acids including six (in vertebrates) to 8 conserved cysteine residues.
Dendritic cell	Dendritic cells are immune cells that form part of the mammalian immune system. Their main function is to process antigen material and present it on the surface to other cells of the immune system, thus functioning as antigen-presenting cells. They act as messengers between the innate and adaptive immunity. Dendritic cells are present in small quantities in tissues that are in contact with the external environment, mainly the skin (where there is a specialized Dendritic cell type called Langerhans cells) and the inner lining of the nose, lungs, stomach and intestines. They can also be found in an immature state in the blood.

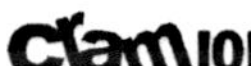

Glucocorticoid	Glucocorticoids are a class of steroid hormones that bind to the Glucocorticoid receptor (GR), which is present in almost every vertebrate animal cell. The name Glucocorticoid derives from their role in the regulation of the metabolism of glucose, their synthesis in the adrenal cortex, and their steroidal structure . GCs are part of the feedback mechanism in the immune system that turns immune activity (inflammation) down.
Leukemia inhibitory factor	Leukemia inhibitory factor, an interleukin 6 class cytokine, is a chemical in cells that affects their growth and development. Leukemia inhibitory factor derives its name from its ability to induce the terminal differentiation of myeloid leukaemic cells. Other properties attributed to the cytokine include: the growth promotion and cell differentiation of different types of target cells, influence on bone metabolism, cachexia, neural development, embryogenesis and inflammation.
Subclinical infection	A Subclinical infection is the asymptomatic (without apparent sign) carrying of an (infection) by an individual of an agent (microbe, intestinal parasite,) that usually is a pathogen causing illness, at least in some individuals. Many pathogens spread by being silently carried in this way by some of their host population. Such infections occur both in humans and nonhuman animals.
Atopy	Atopy or atopic syndrome is an allergic hypersensitivity affecting parts of the body not in direct contact with the allergen. It may involve eczema , allergic conjunctivitis, allergic rhinitis and asthma. There appears to be a strong hereditary component.
Adolescence	Adolescence is a transitional stage of physical and mental human development that occurs between childhood and adulthood. This transition involves biological (i.e. pubertal), social, and psychological changes, though the biological or physiological ones are the easiest to measure objectively. Historically, puberty has been heavily associated with teenagers and the onset of adolescent development.
Sensitization	Sensitization is an example of non-associative learning in which the progressive amplification of a response follows repeated administrations of a stimulus. An everyday example of this mechanism is the repeated tonic stimulation of peripheral nerves that will occur if a person rubs his arm continuously. After a while, this stimulation will create a warm sensation that will eventually turn painful.

Military psychiatrist	A Military psychiatrist is usually a professional that deals with the treatment of military personnel and officers studying the psychological problems consequent to a real war, a virtual one, Treatment and Strategy Counselling. Notable Military psychiatrists are or have been: · Sidney Gottlieb (1918-1999) · Werner Heyde (1902-1964) · Friedrich Panse (1899-1973) · W. H. R. Rivers (1864-1922) · Ernst Rüdin (1874-1952) · Simon Wessely (?-living) `
Bronchial hyperresponsiveness	Bronchial hyperresponsiveness (or other combinations with airway or hyperreactivity) is a state characterised by easily triggered bronchospasm (contraction of the bronchioles or small airways). Bronchial hyperresponsiveness can be assessed with a bronchial challenge test. This most often uses products like metacholine or histamine.
Constipation	Constipation, costiveness,) experiences hard feces (faeces) that are difficult to expel. This usually happens because the colon absorbs too much water from the food. If the food moves through the gastro-intestinal tract too slowly, the colon may absorb too much water, resulting in feces that are dry and hard.

Chapter 2. Physiology and Pathology of Asthma and COPD

Asthma	Asthma is characterized by a predisposition to chronic inflammation of the lungs in which the airways (bronchi) are reversibly narrowed. Asthma affects 7% of the population of the United States, 6.5% of British people and a total of 300 million worldwide. During Asthma attacks (exacerbations of Asthma), the smooth muscle cells in the bronchi constrict, the airways become inflamed and swollen, and breathing becomes difficult.
Epidemic	In epidemiology, an Epidemic occurs when new cases of a certain disease, in a given human population, and during a given period, substantially exceed what is `expected,` based on recent experience . (An epizootic is the analogous circumstance within an animal population). In recent usages, the disease is not required to be communicable; examples include cancer or heart disease.
Factor XII	Hageman factor is a plasma protein , an enzyme (EC 3.4.21.38) of the serine protease (or serine endopeptidase) class. In humans, Factor XII is encoded by the F12 gene. It is part of the coagulation cascade and activates factor XI and prekallikrein.
Functional residual capacity	Functional residual capacity is the volume of air present in the lungs at the end of passive expiration. At Functional residual capacity, the elastic recoil forces of the lungs and chest wall are equal but opposite and there is no exertion by the diaphragm or other respiratory muscles. FRC is the sum of Expiratory Reserve Volume (ERV) and Residual Volume (RV) and measures approximately 2400 ml in a 70 kg, average-sized male.
Lung	The Lung or pulmonary system is the essential respiration organ in all air-breathing animals, including most tetrapods, a few fish and a few snails. In mammals and the more complex life forms, the two Lungs are located in the chest on either side of the heart. Their principal function is to transport oxygen from the atmosphere into the bloodstream, and to release carbon dioxide from the bloodstream into the atmosphere.
Necrosis	Necrosis is the premature death of cells and living tissue. Necrosis is caused by factors external to the cell or tissue, such as infection, toxins, or trauma. This is in contrast to apoptosis, which is a naturally occurring cause of cellular death.
Volume	The Volume of any solid, liquid, gas, plasma, or vacuum is how much three-dimensional space it occupies, often quantified numerically. One-dimensional figures (such as lines) and two-dimensional shapes (such as squares) are assigned zero Volume in the three-dimensional space. Volume is commonly presented in units such as cubic meters, cubic centimeters, liters, or milliliters.

Ehlers-Danlos syndrome	Ehlers-Danlos syndrome is a group of inherited connective tissue disorders, caused by a defect in the synthesis of collagen (a protein in connective tissue). The collagen in connective tissue helps tissues to resist deformation (decreases its elasticity). In the skin, muscles, ligaments, blood vessels, and visceral organs collagen plays a very significant role and with increased elasticity, secondary to abnormal collagen, pathology results.
Elastic recoil	Elastic recoil is the rebound of the lungs after having been stretched by inhalation, or rather, the ease with which the lung rebounds. With inhalation, the interpleural pressure (the pressure within the pleural cavity) of the lungs decreases. Relaxing the diaphragm during expiration allows the lungs to recoil and regain the interpleural pressure experienced previously at rest.
Growth factor	A Growth factor is a naturally occurring substance capable of stimulating cellular growth, proliferation and cellular differentiation. Usually it is a protein or a steroid hormone. Growth factors are important for regulating a variety of cellular processes.
Leukocytes	White blood cells are cells of the immune system defending the body against both infectious disease and foreign materials. Five different and diverse types of Leukocytes exist, but they are all produced and derived from a multipotent cell in the bone marrow known as a hematopoietic stem cell. Leukocytes are found throughout the body, including the blood and lymphatic system.
Neuroendocrine	Neuroendocrine [IPA nÊŠÉ™roÊŠËˆÉ›ndÉ™krÉªn] cells are cells that release a hormone into the circulating blood in response to a neural stimulus. These hormones may be amines, neuropeptides, or specialized amino acids. They package the hormones in vesicles and send these packages via long processes to blood vessels.
Pathology	Pathology is the study and diagnosis of disease through examination of organs, tissues, bodily fluids, and whole bodies (autopsies). The term also encompasses the related scientific study of disease processes, called General Pathology. Medical Pathology is divided in two main branches, Anatomical Pathology and Clinical Pathology.
Artery	The arterial system is the higher-pressure portion of the circulatory system. Arterial pressure varies between the peak pressure during heart contraction, called the systolic pressure, and the minimum, or diastolic pressure between contractions, when the heart expands and refills. This pressure variation within the Artery produces the pulse which is observable in any Artery, and reflects heart activity.

Chronic obstructive pulmonary disease	Chronic obstructive pulmonary disease refers to chronic bronchitis and emphysema, a pair of two commonly co-existing diseases of the lungs in which the airways become narrowed. This leads to a limitation of the flow of air to and from the lungs causing shortness of breath. In contrast to asthma, the limitation of airflow is poorly reversible and usually gets progressively worse over time.
Coronary artery disease	(Coronary artery disease or atherosclerotic heart disease) is the end result of the accumulation of atheromatous plaques within the walls of the coronary arteries that supply the myocardium (the muscle of the heart) with oxygen and nutrients. It is sometimes also called coronary heart disease (CHD), although Coronary artery disease is the most common cause of CHD, it is not the only one. Coronary artery disease is the leading cause of death worldwide.
Coupling	In electronics and telecommunication, coupling is the desirable or undesirable transfer of energy from one medium, such as a metallic wire or an optical fiber, to another medium, including fortuitous transfer. Coupling is also the transfer of electrical energy from one circuit segment to another. For example, energy is transferred from a power source to an electrical load by means of conductive coupling, which may be either resistive or hard-wire. An AC potential may be transferred from one circuit segment to another having a DC potential by use of a capacitor. Electrical energy may be transferred from one circuit segmant to another segment with different impedance by use of a transformer.
Bronchodilator	A Bronchodilator is a substance that dilates the bronchi and bronchioles, decreasing airway resistance and thereby facilitating airflow. Bronchodilators may be endogenous (originating naturally within the body), or they may be medications administered for the treatment of breathing difficulties. They are most useful in obstructive lung diseases, of which asthma and chronic obstructive pulmonary disease are the most common conditions.

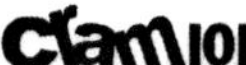

Dose	A dose is a quantity of something (chemical, physical, or biological) that may impact an organism biologically; the greater the quantity, the larger the dose. In nutrition, the term is usually applied to how much of a specific nutrient is in a person's diet or in a particular food, meal, or dietary supplement. In medicine, the term is usually applied to the quantity of a drug or other agent administered for therapeutic purposes.
Gas exchange	Gas exchange takes place at a respiratory surface--a boundary between the external environment and the interior of the organism. For unicellular organisms the respiratory surface is governed by Fick`s law, which determines that respiratory surfaces must have: · a large surface area · a thin permeable surface · a moist exchange surface. Many also have a mechanism to maximise the diffusion gradient by replenishing the source and/or sink. Control of respiration is due to rhythmical breathing generated by the phrenic nerve in order to stimulate contraction and relaxation of the diaphragm during inspiration and expiration.
Vascular endothelial growth factor	Vascular endothelial growth factor is a signal protein produced by cells that stimulates the growth of new blood vessels. It is part of the system that restores the oxygen supply to tissues when blood circulation is inadequate. Vascular endothelial growth factor's normal function is to create new blood vessels during embryonic development, new blood vessels after injury, muscle following exercise, and new vessels (collateral circulation) to bypass blocked vessels.
Matrix	The hair matrix produces the actual hair shaft as well as the inner and outer root sheaths.

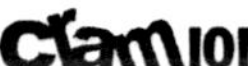

Multiple inert gas elimination technique	Multiple inert gas elimination technique is a technique used mainly in pneumology, that involves measuring mixed venous, arterial, and mixed expired concentrations of six infused inert gases, shows a shunt, dead space, and the general ventilation versus blood flow (Va/Q). It is a good technique for establishing emphysema or chronic bronchitis. `.
Lymphocyte	A Lymphocyte is a type of white blood cell in the vertebrate immune system. Under the microscope, Lymphocytes can be divided into large granular Lymphocytes and small Lymphocytes. Large granular Lymphocytes include natural killer cells (NK cells).
Paracetamol	Paracetamol or acetaminophen) is a widely used over-the-counter analgesic (pain reliever) and antipyretic (fever reducer). However, its effectiveness alone as an antipyretic has been questioned. It is commonly used for the relief of headaches, and other minor aches and pains, and is a major ingredient in numerous cold and flu remedies.
Bronchitis	Bronchitis is inflammation of the mucous membranes of the bronchi, the airways that carry airflow from the trachea into the lungs. Bronchitis can be classified into two categories, acute and chronic, each of which has unique etiologies, pathologies, and therapies. Acute Bronchitis is characterized by the development of a cough, with or without the production of sputum, mucus that is expectorated (coughed up) from the respiratory tract.
Chronic bronchitis	Chronic bronchitis is a chronic inflammation of the bronchi (medium-size airways) in the lungs. It is generally considered one of the two forms of chronic obstructive pulmonary disease (COPD). It is defined clinically as a persistent cough that produces sputum (phlegm) and mucus, for at least three months in two consecutive years.
Emphysema	Emphysema is a lung disease, characterized by an abnormal, permanent enlargement of air spaces distal to the terminal bronchioles. The disease is coupled with the destruction of walls, but without obvious fibrosis. It is often caused by exposure to toxic chemicals, including long-term exposure to tobacco smoke.
Merozoite surface protein	A Merozoite surface protein is a protein molecule taken from the skin, of a merozoite. A merozoite is a \`daughter cell\` of a protozoan. Merozoite surface proteins, or Merozoite surface proteins, are useful in researching malaria, a disease caused by protozoans.

Bronchoalveolar lavage	Bronchoalveolar lavage (BAL) is a medical procedure in which a bronchoscope is passed through the mouth or nose into the lungs and fluid is squirted into a small part of the lung and then recollected for examination. BAL is typically performed to diagnose lung disease. In particular, BAL is commonly used to diagnose infections in people with immune system problems, pneumonia in people on ventilators, some types of lung cancer, and scarring of the lung (interstitial lung disease).
Fibroblast	A Fibroblast is a type of cell that synthesizes the extracellular matrix and collagen, the structural framework (stroma) for animal tissues, and plays a critical role in wound healing. Fibroblasts are the most common cells of connective tissue in animals. Fibroblasts and fibrocytes are two states of the same cells, the former being the activated state, the latter the less active state, concerned with maintenance.
Insulin-like growth factors	The Insulin-like growth factors (Insulin-like growth factorss) are polypeptides with high sequence similarity to insulin. Insulin-like growth factorss are part of a complex system that cells use to communicate with their physiologic environment. This complex system (often referred to as the Insulin-like growth factors `axis`) consists of two cell-surface receptors (Insulin-like growth factors1R and Insulin-like growth factors2R), two ligands (Insulin-like growth factors-1 and Insulin-like growth factors-2), a family of six high-affinity Insulin-like growth factors binding proteins (Insulin-like growth factorsBP 1-6), as well as associated Insulin-like growth factorsBP degrading enzymes, referred to collectively as proteases.
Protein	Proteins are organic compounds made of amino acids arranged in a linear chain and folded into a globular form. The amino acids in a polymer chain are joined together by the peptide bonds between the carboxyl and amino groups of adjacent amino acid residues. The sequence of amino acids in a protein is defined by the sequence of a gene, which is encoded in the genetic code.
Disease	A disease or medical condition is an abnormal condition of an organism that impairs bodily functions, associated with specific symptoms and signs. It may be caused by external factors, such as invading organisms, or it may be caused by internal dysfunctions, such as autoimmune diseases. In human beings, `disease` is often used more broadly to refer to any condition that causes pain, dysfunction, distress, social problems, and/or death to the person afflicted, or similar problems for those in contact with the person.
Obstructive Lung Disease	Obstructive lung disease is a category of respiratory disease characterized by airway obstruction.

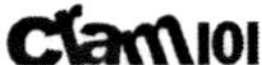

MeSH includes the following in this category:

· Asthma

· Bronchitis

· Chronic obstructive pulmonary disease

Cystic fibrosis is sometimes also included in this category.

FEV1/FVC ratio is usually decreased.

Bone

Bones are rigid organs that form part of the endoskeleton of vertebrates. They function to move, support, and protect the various organs of the body, produce red and white blood cells and store minerals. bone tissue is a type of dense connective tissue.

Corticosteroid

Corticosteroids are a class of steroid hormones that are produced in the adrenal cortex. Corticosteroids are involved in a wide range of physiologic systems such as stress response, immune response and regulation of inflammation, carbohydrate metabolism, protein catabolism, blood electrolyte levels, and behavior.

· Glucocorticoids such as cortisol control carbohydrate, fat and protein metabolism and are anti-inflammatory by preventing phospholipid release, decreasing eosinophil action and a number of other mechanisms.

· Mineralocorticoids such as aldosterone control electrolyte and water levels, mainly by promoting sodium retention in the kidney.

Some common natural hormones are corticosterone ($C_{21}H_{30}O_4$), cortisone ($C_{21}H_{28}O_5$, 17-hydroxy-11-dehydrocorticosterone) and aldosterone.

Granulocytes	Granulocytes are a category of white blood cells characterised by the presence of granules in their cytoplasm. They are also called polymorphonuclear leukocytes (PMN or PML) because of the varying shapes of the nucleus, which is usually lobed into three segments. In common parlance, the term polymorphonuclear leukocyte often refers specifically to neutrophil Granulocytes, the most abundant of the Granulocytes.
Heparin	Heparin, a highly-sulfated glycosaminoglycan, is widely used as an injectable anticoagulant, and has the highest negative charge density of any known biological molecule. It can also be used to form an inner anticoagulant surface on various experimental and medical devices such as test tubes and renal dialysis machines. Pharmaceutical grade Heparin is derived from mucosal tissues of slaughtered meat animals such as porcine (pig) intestine or bovine (cow) lung.
Keratinocyte	Keratinocytes are the predominant cell type in the epidermis, the outermost layer of the human skin, constituting 95% of the cells found there. Those keratinocytes found in the basal layer (Stratum germinativum) of the skin are sometimes referred to as "basal cells" or "basal keratinocytes". The primary function of keratinocytes is the formation of a barrier against environmental damage such as pathogens (bacteria, fungi, parasites, viruses) heat, UV radiation and water loss.
Macrophages	Macrophages are white blood cells within tissues, produced by the division of monocytes. Human Macrophages are about 21 micrometres (0.00083 in) in diameter. Monocytes and Macrophages are phagocytes, acting in both non-specific defense (innate immunity) as well as to help initiate specific defense mechanisms (adaptive immunity) of vertebrate animals.
Metabolism	Metabolism is the set of chemical reactions that happen in living organisms to maintain life. These processes allow organisms to grow and reproduce, maintain their structures, and respond to their environments. Metabolism is usually divided into two categories.
Basement membrane	The Basement membrane is a thin sheet of fibers that underlies the epithelium, which lines the cavities and surfaces of organs, or the endothelium, which lines the interior surface of blood vessels. The Basement membrane is the fusion of two basal laminae. It consists of an electron-dense membrane called the lamina densa, about 30-70 nanometers in thickness, and an underlying network of reticular collagen (type III) fibrils (its precursor is fibroblasts) which average 30 nanometers in diameter and 0.1-2 micrometers in thickness.
Colitis	Colitis is a chronic digestive disease characterized by inflammation of the colon.

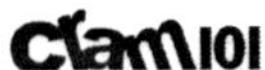

	Colitis is one of a group of conditions which are inflammatory and auto-immune, affecting the tissue that lines the gastrointestinal system (the large and small intestine). It is classed as an inflammatory bowel disease (IBD), not to be confused with irritable bowel syndrome (IBS).
Ulcerative colitis	Ulcerative colitis (Colitis ulcerosa, Ulcerative colitis) is a form of inflammatory bowel disease (IBD). Ulcerative colitis is a form of colitis, a disease of the intestine, specifically the large intestine or colon, that includes characteristic ulcers, or open sores, in the colon. The main symptom of active disease is usually constant diarrhea mixed with blood, of gradual onset.
Usual interstitial pneumonia	Usual interstitial pneumonia, commonly abbreviated Usual interstitial pneumonia, is the name of a histopathological pattern seen in diffuse lung diseases, i.e. interstitial lung diseases. It is classified as an idiopathic interstitial pneumonia, and may be idiopathic, i.e. the cause is unknown, or due to a known cause, e.g. asbestos exposure. The hallmarks of Usual interstitial pneumonia are interstitial inflammation, i.e. inflammation of the alveolar walls, and fibrosis (scarring).
Constipation	Constipation, costiveness,) experiences hard feces (faeces) that are difficult to expel. This usually happens because the colon absorbs too much water from the food. If the food moves through the gastro-intestinal tract too slowly, the colon may absorb too much water, resulting in feces that are dry and hard.
Positive end-expiratory pressure	Positive end-expiratory pressure (PEEP) is a term used in mechanical ventilation to denote the amount of pressure above atmospheric pressure present in the airway at the end of the expiratory cycle. The equivalent in a spontaneously breathing patient is CPAP. PEEP is set on the ventilator. PEEP improves gas exchange by preventing alveolar collapse, recruiting more lung units, increasing functional residual capacity, and redistributing fluid in the alveoli.
Glucocorticoid	Glucocorticoids are a class of steroid hormones that bind to the Glucocorticoid receptor (GR), which is present in almost every vertebrate animal cell. The name Glucocorticoid derives from their role in the regulation of the metabolism of glucose, their synthesis in the adrenal cortex, and their steroidal structure . GCs are part of the feedback mechanism in the immune system that turns immune activity (inflammation) down.

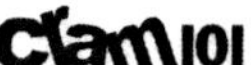

Omalizumab	Omalizumab (Xolair, Genentech / Novartis) is a humanized antibody drug approved for patients with moderate-to-severe or severe allergic asthma, which is caused by hypersensitivity reactions to certain harmless environmental substances. Omalizumab`s cost is high ($10,000 to $30,000 per year), as compared to other drugs used for asthma, and hence Omalizumab is mainly prescribed for patients with severe, persistent asthma, which cannot be controlled even with high doses of corticosteroids. Like other protein and antibody drugs, Omalizumab causes anaphylaxis (a life-threatening systemic allergic reaction) in 1 to 2 patients per 1,000.

Marfan syndrome	Marfan syndrome is a genetic disorder of the connective tissue. It is sometimes inherited as a dominant trait. It is carried by a gene called FBN1, which encodes a connective protein called fibrillin-1. People have a pair of FBN1 genes.
Bronchoalveolar lavage	Bronchoalveolar lavage (BAL) is a medical procedure in which a bronchoscope is passed through the mouth or nose into the lungs and fluid is squirted into a small part of the lung and then recollected for examination. BAL is typically performed to diagnose lung disease. In particular, BAL is commonly used to diagnose infections in people with immune system problems, pneumonia in people on ventilators, some types of lung cancer, and scarring of the lung (interstitial lung disease).
Factor XII	Hageman factor is a plasma protein , an enzyme (EC 3.4.21.38) of the serine protease (or serine endopeptidase) class. In humans, Factor XII is encoded by the F12 gene. It is part of the coagulation cascade and activates factor XI and prekallikrein.
Fibroblast	A Fibroblast is a type of cell that synthesizes the extracellular matrix and collagen, the structural framework (stroma) for animal tissues, and plays a critical role in wound healing. Fibroblasts are the most common cells of connective tissue in animals. Fibroblasts and fibrocytes are two states of the same cells, the former being the activated state, the latter the less active state, concerned with maintenance.
Growth factor	A Growth factor is a naturally occurring substance capable of stimulating cellular growth, proliferation and cellular differentiation. Usually it is a protein or a steroid hormone. Growth factors are important for regulating a variety of cellular processes.
Mast cell	A Mast cell is a resident cell of several types of tissues and contains many granules rich in histamine and heparin. Although best known for their role in allergy and anaphylaxis, Mast cells play an important protective role as well, being intimately involved in wound healing and defense against pathogens. Mast cells were first described by Paul Ehrlich in his 1878 doctoral thesis on the basis of their unique staining characteristics and large granules.

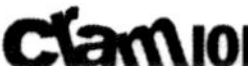

Asthma	Asthma is characterized by a predisposition to chronic inflammation of the lungs in which the airways (bronchi) are reversibly narrowed. Asthma affects 7% of the population of the United States, 6.5% of British people and a total of 300 million worldwide. During Asthma attacks (exacerbations of Asthma), the smooth muscle cells in the bronchi constrict, the airways become inflamed and swollen, and breathing becomes difficult.
Artery	The arterial system is the higher-pressure portion of the circulatory system. Arterial pressure varies between the peak pressure during heart contraction, called the systolic pressure, and the minimum, or diastolic pressure between contractions, when the heart expands and refills. This pressure variation within the Artery produces the pulse which is observable in any Artery, and reflects heart activity.
Paracetamol	Paracetamol or acetaminophen) is a widely used over-the-counter analgesic (pain reliever) and antipyretic (fever reducer). However, its effectiveness alone as an antipyretic has been questioned. It is commonly used for the relief of headaches, and other minor aches and pains, and is a major ingredient in numerous cold and flu remedies.
Ehlers-Danlos syndrome	Ehlers-Danlos syndrome is a group of inherited connective tissue disorders, caused by a defect in the synthesis of collagen (a protein in connective tissue). The collagen in connective tissue helps tissues to resist deformation (decreases its elasticity). In the skin, muscles, ligaments, blood vessels, and visceral organs collagen plays a very significant role and with increased elasticity, secondary to abnormal collagen, pathology results.
Cystic fibrosis	Cystic fibrosis (also known as Cystic fibrosis, mucovoidosis,) is a genetic disorder known to be an inherited disease of the secretory glands, including the glands that make mucus and sweat. The hallmarks of Cystic fibrosis are salty tasting skin, normal appetite but poor growth and poor weight gain, excess mucus production, frequent chest infections and coughing/shortness of breath. Males can be infertile due to the condition Congenital absence of the vas deferens.
Leukocytes	White blood cells are cells of the immune system defending the body against both infectious disease and foreign materials. Five different and diverse types of Leukocytes exist, but they are all produced and derived from a multipotent cell in the bone marrow known as a hematopoietic stem cell. Leukocytes are found throughout the body, including the blood and lymphatic system.

Chronic obstructive pulmonary disease	Chronic obstructive pulmonary disease refers to chronic bronchitis and emphysema, a pair of two commonly co-existing diseases of the lungs in which the airways become narrowed. This leads to a limitation of the flow of air to and from the lungs causing shortness of breath. In contrast to asthma, the limitation of airflow is poorly reversible and usually gets progressively worse over time.
Coronary artery disease	(Coronary artery disease or atherosclerotic heart disease) is the end result of the accumulation of atheromatous plaques within the walls of the coronary arteries that supply the myocardium (the muscle of the heart) with oxygen and nutrients. It is sometimes also called coronary heart disease (CHD), although Coronary artery disease is the most common cause of CHD, it is not the only one. Coronary artery disease is the leading cause of death worldwide.
Corticosteroid	Corticosteroids are a class of steroid hormones that are produced in the adrenal cortex. Corticosteroids are involved in a wide range of physiologic systems such as stress response, immune response and regulation of inflammation, carbohydrate metabolism, protein catabolism, blood electrolyte levels, and behavior. · Glucocorticoids such as cortisol control carbohydrate, fat and protein metabolism and are anti-inflammatory by preventing phospholipid release, decreasing eosinophil action and a number of other mechanisms. · Mineralocorticoids such as aldosterone control electrolyte and water levels, mainly by promoting sodium retention in the kidney. Some common natural hormones are corticosterone ($C_{21}H_{30}O_4$), cortisone ($C_{21}H_{28}O_5$, 17-hydroxy-11-dehydrocorticosterone) and aldosterone.

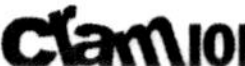

Chapter 3. Inflammatory Cells and Extracellular Matrix

Heparin	Heparin, a highly-sulfated glycosaminoglycan, is widely used as an injectable anticoagulant, and has the highest negative charge density of any known biological molecule. It can also be used to form an inner anticoagulant surface on various experimental and medical devices such as test tubes and renal dialysis machines. Pharmaceutical grade Heparin is derived from mucosal tissues of slaughtered meat animals such as porcine (pig) intestine or bovine (cow) lung.
Defensins	Defensins are small cysteine-rich cationic proteins found in both vertebrates and invertebrates. They are active against bacteria, fungi and many enveloped and nonenveloped viruses. They consist of 18-45 amino acids including six (in vertebrates) to 8 conserved cysteine residues.
Dendritic cell	Dendritic cells are immune cells that form part of the mammalian immune system. Their main function is to process antigen material and present it on the surface to other cells of the immune system, thus functioning as antigen-presenting cells. They act as messengers between the innate and adaptive immunity. Dendritic cells are present in small quantities in tissues that are in contact with the external environment, mainly the skin (where there is a specialized Dendritic cell type called Langerhans cells) and the inner lining of the nose, lungs, stomach and intestines. They can also be found in an immature state in the blood.
Lung	The Lung or pulmonary system is the essential respiration organ in all air-breathing animals, including most tetrapods, a few fish and a few snails. In mammals and the more complex life forms, the two Lungs are located in the chest on either side of the heart. Their principal function is to transport oxygen from the atmosphere into the bloodstream, and to release carbon dioxide from the bloodstream into the atmosphere.
Volume	The Volume of any solid, liquid, gas, plasma, or vacuum is how much three-dimensional space it occupies, often quantified numerically. One-dimensional figures (such as lines) and two-dimensional shapes (such as squares) are assigned zero Volume in the three-dimensional space. Volume is commonly presented in units such as cubic meters, cubic centimeters, liters, or milliliters.
Mycoplasma pneumonia	Mycoplasma pneumonia is a form of bacterial pneumonia which is caused by the bacteria species Mycoplasma pneumoniae. Disease from mycoplasma is usually mild to moderate in severity. The symptoms are usually mild enough that the patient may remain ambulatory throughout the illness.
Myeloid	The term Myeloid suggests an origin in the bone marrow or spinal cord, or a resemblance to the marrow or spinal cord.

	In hematopoiesis, the term `Myeloid cell` is used to describe any leukocyte that is not a lymphocyte. This terminology is frequently seen when classifying cancers, especially leukemia.
Protein	Proteins are organic compounds made of amino acids arranged in a linear chain and folded into a globular form. The amino acids in a polymer chain are joined together by the peptide bonds between the carboxyl and amino groups of adjacent amino acid residues. The sequence of amino acids in a protein is defined by the sequence of a gene, which is encoded in the genetic code.
Sensitization	Sensitization is an example of non-associative learning in which the progressive amplification of a response follows repeated administrations of a stimulus. An everyday example of this mechanism is the repeated tonic stimulation of peripheral nerves that will occur if a person rubs his arm continuously. After a while, this stimulation will create a warm sensation that will eventually turn painful.
Allergic inflammation	Allergic inflammation is an important pathophysiological feature of several disabilities or medical conditions including allergic asthma, atopic dermatitis, allergic rhinitis and several ocular allergic diseases. Allergic reactions may generally be divided into two components; the early phase reaction, and the late phase reaction. While the contribution to the development of symptoms from each of the phases varies greatly between diseases, both are usually present and provide us a framework for understanding allergic disease .
Granulocytes	Granulocytes are a category of white blood cells characterised by the presence of granules in their cytoplasm. They are also called polymorphonuclear leukocytes (PMN or PML) because of the varying shapes of the nucleus, which is usually lobed into three segments. In common parlance, the term polymorphonuclear leukocyte often refers specifically to neutrophil Granulocytes, the most abundant of the Granulocytes.
Macrophages	Macrophages are white blood cells within tissues, produced by the division of monocytes. Human Macrophages are about 21 micrometres (0.00083 in) in diameter. Monocytes and Macrophages are phagocytes, acting in both non-specific defense (innate immunity) as well as to help initiate specific defense mechanisms (adaptive immunity) of vertebrate animals.
Progressive massive fibrosis	Progressive massive fibrosis is , and then through the body`s immunological reactions to the dust.
Homostatic	The adjective homostatic has been used to refer to homografts which are inert when transplanted into the recipient.

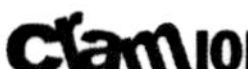

Chapter 3. Inflammatory Cells and Extracellular Matrix

Neuroendocrine	Neuroendocrine [IPA nÊŠÉ™roÊŠËˆÉ›ndÉ™krÉªn] cells are cells that release a hormone into the circulating blood in response to a neural stimulus. These hormones may be amines, neuropeptides, or specialized amino acids. They package the hormones in vesicles and send these packages via long processes to blood vessels.
Antigen-presenting cell	An Antigen-presenting cell or accessory cell is a cell that displays foreign antigen complex with major histocompatibility complex (MHC) on its surface. T-cells may recognize this complex using their T-cell receptor (TCR). These cells process antigens and present them to T-cells.
Immunity	Immunity is a biological term that describes a state of having sufficient biological defenses to avoid infection, disease, or other unwanted biological invasion. Immunity involves both specific and non-specific components. The non-specific components act either as barriers or as eliminators of wide range of pathogens irrespective of antigenic specificity.
Matrix	The hair matrix produces the actual hair shaft as well as the inner and outer root sheaths.
Viral	The term Viral is used to describe anything related to viruses. Viral may also mean: · .
Antigen presentation	Antigen presentation is a process in the body's immune system by which macrophages, dendritic cells and other cell types capture antigens and then enable their recognition by T-cells. The basis of adaptive immunity lies in the capacity of immune cells to distinguish between the body's own cells, and infectious pathogens. The host's cells express 'self' antigens that identify them as such.
Respiratory burst	Respiratory burst (is) is the rapid release of reactive oxygen species (superoxide radical and hydrogen peroxide) from different types of cells.

	Usually it denotes the release of these chemicals from immune cells, e.g., neutrophils and monocytes, as they come into contact with different bacteria or fungi. They are also released from the ovum of higher animals after the ovum has been fertilized.
Interferon	Interferons (IFNs) are proteins made and released by lymphocytes in response to the presence of pathogens--such as viruses, bacteria, or parasites--or tumor cells. They allow communication between cells to trigger the protective defenses of the immune system that eradicate pathogens or tumors. Interferons belong to the large class of glycoproteins known as cytokines.
Monoclonal antibodies	Monoclonal antibodies (mAb or moAb) are monospecific antibodies that are identical because they are produced by one type of immune cell that are all clones of a single parent cell. Given almost any substance, it is possible to create Monoclonal antibodies that specifically bind to that substance; they can then serve to detect or purify that substance. This has become an important tool in biochemistry, molecular biology and medicine.
Lymphocyte	A Lymphocyte is a type of white blood cell in the vertebrate immune system. Under the microscope, Lymphocytes can be divided into large granular Lymphocytes and small Lymphocytes. Large granular Lymphocytes include natural killer cells (NK cells).
Glucocorticoid	Glucocorticoids are a class of steroid hormones that bind to the Glucocorticoid receptor (GR), which is present in almost every vertebrate animal cell. The name Glucocorticoid derives from their role in the regulation of the metabolism of glucose, their synthesis in the adrenal cortex, and their steroidal structure . GCs are part of the feedback mechanism in the immune system that turns immune activity (inflammation) down.
Endogenous	The word Endogenous means 'proceeding from within', the opposite of exogenous. Endogenous substances are those that originate from within an organism, tissue, or cell . Endogenous retrovirus are caused by ancient infections of germ cells in humans, mammals and other vertebrates.

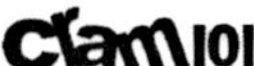

Epithelial-mesenchymal transition	Epithelial-mesenchymal transition is a hypothesized program of development of biological cells characterized by loss of cell adhesion, repression of E-cadherin expression, and increased cell mobility. Epithelial mesenchymal transition may be essential for numerous developmental processes including mesoderm formation and neural tube formation. Induction Several oncogenic pathways (peptide growth factors, Src, Ras, Ets, integrin, Wnt/beta-catenin and Notch) may induce Epithelial mesenchymal transition. In particular, Ras-MAPK has been shown to activate two related transcription factors known as Snail and Slug.
Military psychiatrist	A Military psychiatrist is usually a professional that deals with the treatment of military personnel and officers studying the psychological problems consequent to a real war, a virtual one, Treatment and Strategy Counselling. Notable Military psychiatrists are or have been: · Sidney Gottlieb (1918-1999) · Werner Heyde (1902-1964) · Friedrich Panse (1899-1973) · W. H. R. Rivers (1864-1922) · Ernst Rüdin (1874-1952) · Simon Wessely (?-living) `
Platelet	Platelets, or thrombocytes , are small, irregularly-shaped anuclear cells , 2-3 Âµm in diameter, which are derived from fragmentation of precursor megakaryocytes. The average lifespan of a Platelet is between 8 and 12 days. Platelets play a fundamental role in hemostasis and are a natural source of growth factors.

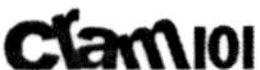

Matrix metalloproteinases	Matrix metalloproteinases are zinc-dependent endopeptidases; other family members are adamalysins, serralysins, and astacins. The MMPs belong to a larger family of proteases known as the metzincin superfamily.
	Collectively they are capable of degrading all kinds of extracellular matrix proteins, but also can process a number of bioactive molecules.
Bronchoscopy	Bronchoscopy is a technique of visualizing the inside of the airways for diagnostic and therapeutic purposes. An instrument (bronchoscope) is inserted into the airways, usually through the nose or mouth, or occasionally through a tracheostomy. This allows the practitioner to examine the patient's airways for abnormalities such as foreign bodies, bleeding, tumors, or inflammation.
Idiopathic	Idiopathic is an adjective used primarily in medicine meaning arising spontaneously or from an obscure or unknown cause. From Greek á¼´διος, idios + πÎ¬θος, pathos (suffering), it means approximately `a disease of its own kind.` It is technically a term from nosology, the classification of disease. For most medical conditions, one or more causes are somewhat understood, but in a certain percentage of people with the condition, the cause may not be readily apparent or characterized.
Idiopathic pulmonary fibrosis	Idiopathic pulmonary fibrosis , formerly known as cryptogenic fibrosing alveolitis, is a rare, chronic, progressive interstitial lung disease. Idiopathic pulmonary fibrosis belongs to the subgroup, known as idiopathic interstitial pneumonia (IIP). It is the most common form of the seven distinct IIPs.
Multiple inert gas elimination technique	Multiple inert gas elimination technique is a technique used mainly in pneumology, that involves measuring mixed venous, arterial, and mixed expired concentrations of six infused inert gases, shows a shunt, dead space, and the general ventilation versus blood flow (Va/Q). It is a good technique for establishing emphysema or chronic bronchitis. `.
Allergen	An Allergen is a nonparasitic antigen capable of stimulating a type-I hypersensitivity reaction in atopic individuals. Most humans mount significant Immunoglobulin E responses only as a defense against parasitic infections. However, some individuals mount an IgE response against common environmental antigens.

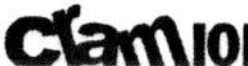

Myofibroblast	A Myofibroblast is a cell that is in between a fibroblast and a smooth muscle cell in differentiation. There are many possible ways of Myofibroblast development: · Partial smooth muscle differentiation of a fibroblastic cell · Activation of a stellate cell (eg Hepatic Ito cells or pancreatic stellate cells). · Loss of contractile phenotype (or acquisition of `synthetic phenotype`) of a smooth muscle cell. · Direct Myofibroblastic differentiation of a progenitor cell resident in a stromal tissue. · Homing and recruitment of a circulating mesenchymal precursor which can directly differentiate as above or indirectly differentiate through the other cell types as intermediates. · Epithelial to mesenchymal transdifferentiation of an epithelial cell. Myofibroblasts usually stain for the intermediate filament vimentin which is a general mesenchymal marker and `alpha smooth muscle actin`. They are positive for other smooth markers like another intermediate filament type desmin positive in some tissues but may be negative for desmin in some others.
Acute respiratory distress syndrome	Acute respiratory distress syndrome , also known as respiratory distress syndrome (RDS) or adult respiratory distress syndrome (in contrast with IRDS) is a serious reaction to various forms of injuries to the lung. Acute respiratory distress syndrome is a severe lung disease caused by a variety of direct and indirect issues. It is characterized by inflammation of the lung parenchyma leading to impaired gas exchange with concomitant systemic release of inflammatory mediators causing inflammation, hypoxemia and frequently resulting in multiple organ failure.
Bleomycin	Bleomycin is a glycopeptide antibiotic produced by the bacterium Streptomyces verticillus. Bleomycin refers to a family of structurally related compounds. When used as an anticancer agent, the chemotherapeutical forms are primarily bleomycin A_2 and B_2.

Chapter 3. Inflammatory Cells and Extracellular Matrix

Coagulation	Coagulation is a complex process by which blood forms clots. It is an important part of hemostasis , wherein a damaged blood vessel wall is covered by a platelet and fibrin-containing clot to stop bleeding and begin repair of the damaged vessel. Disorders of Coagulation can lead to an increased risk of bleeding (hemorrhage) or clotting (thrombosis).
Septa	Each lobule of the testis is contained in one of the intervals between the fibrous septa which extend between the mediastinum testis and the tunica albuginea, and consists of from one to three, minute convoluted tubes, the tubuli seminiferi. .
Pathology	Pathology is the study and diagnosis of disease through examination of organs, tissues, bodily fluids, and whole bodies (autopsies). The term also encompasses the related scientific study of disease processes, called General Pathology. Medical Pathology is divided in two main branches, Anatomical Pathology and Clinical Pathology.
Protease	This article discusses primarily the structure and properties of proteolytic enzymes. For medical, surgical and related applications of several Proteases, see article: Proteases (medical and related uses) Proteases break down proteins. A Protease is any enzyme that conducts proteolysis, that is, begins protein catabolism by hydrolysis of the peptide bonds that link amino acids together in the polypeptide chain, which form a molecule of protein.
Caries	Caries is a progressive destruction of any kind of bone structure, including the skull, ribs and other bones, which is a bacterial disease. A disease that involves Caries is mastoiditis, an inflammation of the mastoid process, in which the bone gets eroded.
Thrombin	Thrombin (activated Factor II [IIa]) also commonly called pro-Thrombin is a coagulation protein in the blood stream that has many effects in the coagulation cascade. It is a serine protease (EC 3.4.21.5) that converts soluble fibrinogen into insoluble strands of fibrin, as well as catalyzing many other coagulation-related reactions. The Thrombin (proThrombin) gene is located on the eleventh chromosome (11p11-q12).
Progenitor cells	Like stem cells, Progenitor cells have a capacity to differentiate into a specific type of cell. In contrast to stem cells, however, they are already far more specific: they are pushed to differentiate into their \`target\` cell. The most important difference between stem cells and Progenitor cells is that stem cells can replicate indefinitely, whereas Progenitor cells can only divide a limited number of times. Progenitor cells are found in adult organisms and they act as a repair system for the body. They replenish special cells, but also maintain the blood, skin and intestinal tissues.

Cladosporium	Cladosporium is a genus of fungi including some of the most common indoor and outdoor molds. It produces olive-green to brown or black colonies, and its dark-pigmented conidia are formed in simple or branching chains. The many species of Cladosporium are commonly found on living and dead plant material.
Clearance	In medicine, the clearance is a measurement of the renal excretion ability. Although clearance may also involve other organs than the kidney, it is almost synonymous with renal clearance or renal plasma clearance. Each substance has a specific clearance that depends on its filtration characteristics.
Dyskinesia	Dyskinesia is a movement disorder which consists of effects including diminished voluntary movements and the presence of involuntary movements, similar to tics or chorea. Dyskinesia is a symptom of several medical disorders and is distinguished by the underlying cause. When a Dyskinesia presents after treatment with an antipsychotic drug such as haloperidol (Haldol), it is known as tardive Dyskinesia, and is commonly seen in the face and mouth in the form of \`tongue rolling\`.
Primary	In medicine, the reporting of symptoms by a patient may have significant psychological motivators. Psychologists sometimes categorize these motivators into primary or secondary gain. primary gain is internally good; motivationally.
Immune system	An Immune system is a system of biological structures and processes within an organism that protects against disease by identifying and killing pathogens and tumor cells. It detects a wide variety of agents, from viruses to parasitic worms, and needs to distinguish them from the organism\`s own healthy cells and tissues in order to function properly. Detection is complicated as pathogens can evolve rapidly, producing adaptations that avoid the Immune system and allow the pathogens to successfully infect their hosts.
Monitoring	To monitor or Monitoring generally means to be aware of the state of a system. Below are specific examples: · to observe a situation for any changes which may occur over time, using a monitor or measuring device of some sort: · Baby monitor, medical monitor, Heart rate monitor

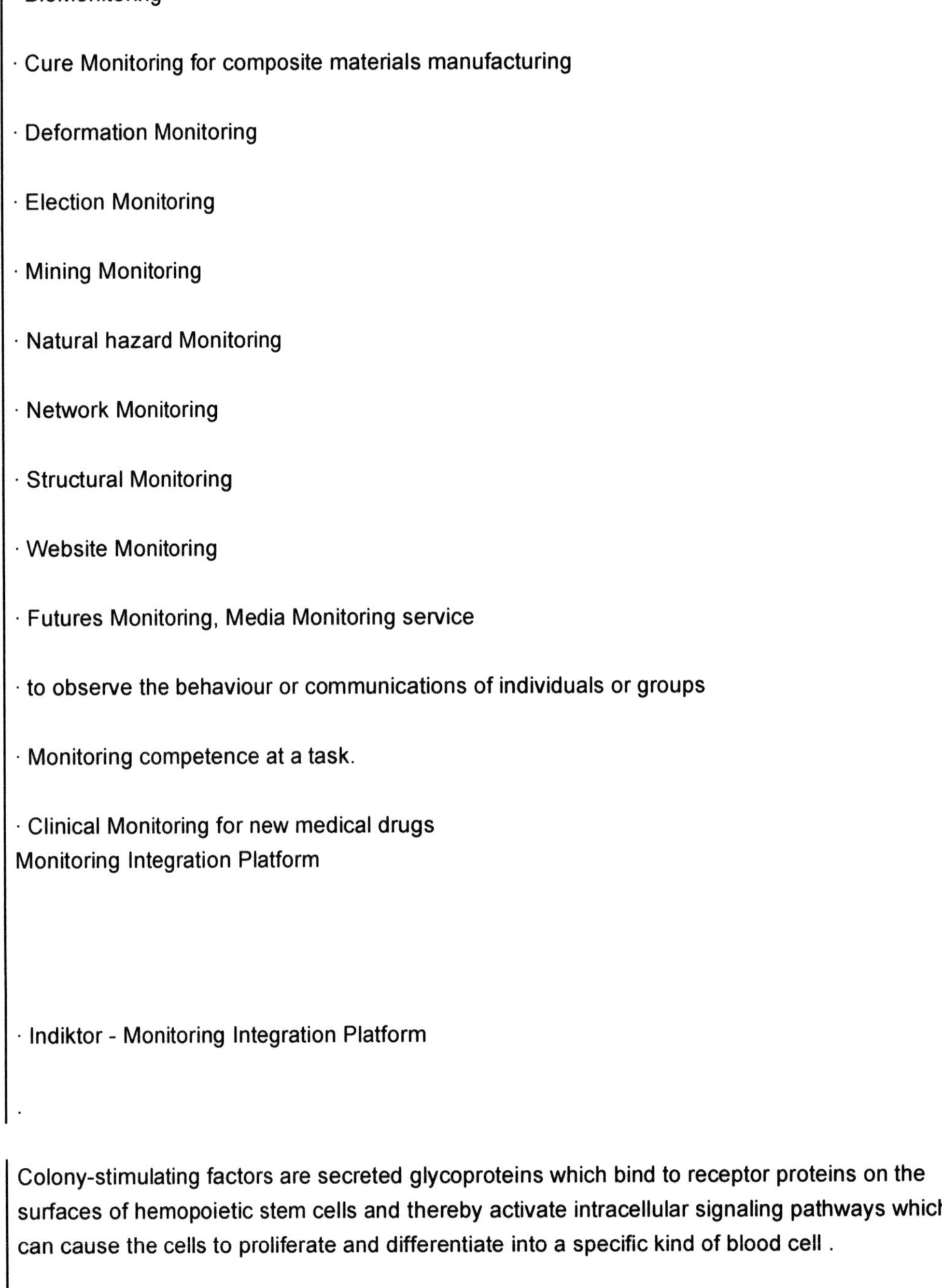

· BioMonitoring

· Cure Monitoring for composite materials manufacturing

· Deformation Monitoring

· Election Monitoring

· Mining Monitoring

· Natural hazard Monitoring

· Network Monitoring

· Structural Monitoring

· Website Monitoring

· Futures Monitoring, Media Monitoring service

· to observe the behaviour or communications of individuals or groups

· Monitoring competence at a task.

· Clinical Monitoring for new medical drugs
Monitoring Integration Platform

· Indiktor - Monitoring Integration Platform

·

Colony-stimulating factor	Colony-stimulating factors are secreted glycoproteins which bind to receptor proteins on the surfaces of hemopoietic stem cells and thereby activate intracellular signaling pathways which can cause the cells to proliferate and differentiate into a specific kind of blood cell .

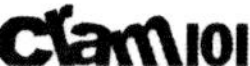

	They may be synthesized and administered exogenously. However, such molecules can at a latter stage be detected, since they differ slightly from the endogenous ones in e.g.
Granulocyte-macrophage colony-stimulating factor	Granulocyte-macrophage colony-stimulating factor, often abbreviated to GM-CSF, is a protein secreted by macrophages, T cells, mast cells, endothelial cells and fibroblasts. GM-CSF is a cytokine that functions as a white blood cell growth factor. GM-CSF stimulates stem cells to produce granulocytes and monocytes.
Bronchitis	Bronchitis is inflammation of the mucous membranes of the bronchi, the airways that carry airflow from the trachea into the lungs. Bronchitis can be classified into two categories, acute and chronic, each of which has unique etiologies, pathologies, and therapies. Acute Bronchitis is characterized by the development of a cough, with or without the production of sputum, mucus that is expectorated (coughed up) from the respiratory tract.
Status asthmaticus	Status asthmaticus is an acute exacerbation of asthma that does not respond to standard treatments of bronchodilators and corticosteroids. Symptoms include chest tightness, rapidly progressive dyspnea (shortness of breath), dry cough, use of accessory muscles, labored breathing and extreme wheezing. It is a life-threatening episode of airway obstruction considered a medical emergency.
Disease	A disease or medical condition is an abnormal condition of an organism that impairs bodily functions, associated with specific symptoms and signs. It may be caused by external factors, such as invading organisms, or it may be caused by internal dysfunctions, such as autoimmune diseases. In human beings, `disease` is often used more broadly to refer to any condition that causes pain, dysfunction, distress, social problems, and/or death to the person afflicted, or similar problems for those in contact with the person.
Obstructive Lung Disease	Obstructive lung disease is a category of respiratory disease characterized by airway obstruction. MeSH includes the following in this category: · Asthma · Bronchitis

· Chronic obstructive pulmonary disease
Cystic fibrosis is sometimes also included in this category.

FEV1/FVC ratio is usually decreased.

SNARE

SNARE proteins REceptors` are a large protein superfamily consisting of more than 60 members in yeast and mammalian cells.
The primary role of SNARE proteins is to mediate vesicle fusion, that is, the exocytosis of cellular transport vesicles with the cell membrane at the porosome or with a target compartment (such as a lysosome).

SNAREs can be divided into two categories: vesicle or v-SNAREs , which are incorporated into the membranes of transport vesicles during budding, and target or t-SNAREs, which are located in the membranes of target compartments.

Calcium channel

A Calcium channel is an ion channel which displays selective permeabiltiy to calcium ions. It is sometimes synonymous as voltage-dependent calcium channel, although there are also ligand-gated calcium channels.

Comparison tables

The following tables explain gating, gene, location and function of different types of calcium channels, both voltage and ligand-gated.

Ejection fraction

In cardiovascular physiology, ejection fraction is the fraction of blood pumped out of the right and left ventricles with each heart beat. The term ejection fraction applies to both the right and left ventricles; one can speak equally of the left ventricular ejection fraction and the right ventricular ejection fraction. RVEF and LVEF may vary widely from one another incumbent upon physiologic state.

Allostasis

Allostasis is the process of achieving stability, through physiological or behavioral change. This can be carried out by means of alteration in HPA axis hormones, the autonomic nervous system, cytokines, or a number of other systems, and is generally adaptive in the short term Allostasis is essential in order to maintain internal viability amid changing conditions (Sterling and Eyer, 1988; McEwen, 1998a, 1998b; Schulkin, 2003).

	The concept of Allostasis was proposed by Sterling and Eyer in 1988 to describe an additional process of reestablishing homeostasis, but one that responds to a challenge instead of to subtle ebb and flow.
Necrosis	Necrosis is the premature death of cells and living tissue. Necrosis is caused by factors external to the cell or tissue, such as infection, toxins, or trauma. This is in contrast to apoptosis, which is a naturally occurring cause of cellular death.
Salbutamol	Salbutamol (INN) or albuterol (USAN) is a short-acting β_2-adrenergic receptor agonist used for the relief of bronchospasm in conditions such as asthma and chronic obstructive pulmonary disease. It is marketed by GlaxoSmithKline as Ventolin, Aerolin or Ventorlin depending on the market; by Cipla as Asthalin; by Schering-Plough as Proventil and by Teva as ProAir. Generic names are currently not available in the U.S. because of a federal ban on the use of CFCs.
Subclinical infection	A Subclinical infection is the asymptomatic (without apparent sign) carrying of an (infection) by an individual of an agent (microbe, intestinal parasite,) that usually is a pathogen causing illness, at least in some individuals. Many pathogens spread by being silently carried in this way by some of their host population. Such infections occur both in humans and nonhuman animals.
Bone	Bones are rigid organs that form part of the endoskeleton of vertebrates. They function to move, support, and protect the various organs of the body, produce red and white blood cells and store minerals. bone tissue is a type of dense connective tissue.
Fenoterol	Fenoterol is an asthma medication designed to open up the airways to the lungs. It is classed as a beta agonist. Fenoterol was marketed as `Berotec` by Boehringer-Ingelheim.
Metabolism	Metabolism is the set of chemical reactions that happen in living organisms to maintain life. These processes allow organisms to grow and reproduce, maintain their structures, and respond to their environments. Metabolism is usually divided into two categories.
Colitis	Colitis is a chronic digestive disease characterized by inflammation of the colon. Colitis is one of a group of conditions which are inflammatory and auto-immune, affecting the tissue that lines the gastrointestinal system (the large and small intestine). It is classed as an inflammatory bowel disease (IBD), not to be confused with irritable bowel syndrome (IBS).

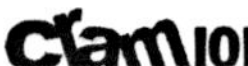

Ulcerative colitis	Ulcerative colitis (Colitis ulcerosa, Ulcerative colitis) is a form of inflammatory bowel disease (IBD). Ulcerative colitis is a form of colitis, a disease of the intestine, specifically the large intestine or colon, that includes characteristic ulcers, or open sores, in the colon. The main symptom of active disease is usually constant diarrhea mixed with blood, of gradual onset.
Usual interstitial pneumonia	Usual interstitial pneumonia, commonly abbreviated Usual interstitial pneumonia, is the name of a histopathological pattern seen in diffuse lung diseases, i.e. interstitial lung diseases. It is classified as an idiopathic interstitial pneumonia, and may be idiopathic, i.e. the cause is unknown, or due to a known cause, e.g. asbestos exposure. The hallmarks of Usual interstitial pneumonia are interstitial inflammation, i.e. inflammation of the alveolar walls, and fibrosis (scarring).
Gas exchange	Gas exchange takes place at a respiratory surface--a boundary between the external environment and the interior of the organism. For unicellular organisms the respiratory surface is governed by Fick`s law, which determines that respiratory surfaces must have: · a large surface area · a thin permeable surface · a moist exchange surface. Many also have a mechanism to maximise the diffusion gradient by replenishing the source and/or sink. Control of respiration is due to rhythmical breathing generated by the phrenic nerve in order to stimulate contraction and relaxation of the diaphragm during inspiration and expiration.
Substance P	In the field of neuroscience, Substance P is a neuropeptide: an undecapeptide that functions as a neurotransmitter and as a neuromodulator. It belongs to the tachykinin neuropeptide family. Substance P and its closely related neuropeptide neurokinin A (NKA) are produced from a polyprotein precursor after differential splicing of the preprotachykinin A gene. The deduced amino acid sequence of Substance P is as follows:

	· Arg Pro Lys Pro Gln Gln Phe Phe Gly Leu Met Substance P is released from the terminals of specific sensory nerves, it is found in the brain and spinal cord, and is associated with inflammatory processes and pain.
Blood flow	Blood flow is the flow of blood in the cardiovascular system. It can be calculated by dividing the vascular resistance into the pressure gradient. Mathematically, Blood flow is described by Darcy's law (which can be viewed as the fluid equivalent of Ohm's law) and approximately by Hagen-Poiseuille equation.
Connective tissue	Connective tissue is a form of fibrous tissue. It is one of the four types of tissue in traditional classifications (the others being epithelial, muscle, and nervous tissue). Collagen is the main protein of Connective tissue in animals and the most abundant protein in mammals, making up about 25% of the total protein content. Fiber types as follows: · collagenous fibers · elastic fibers · Bone Marrow Various Connective tissue conditions have been identified; these can be both inherited and environmental. · Marfan syndrome - a genetic disease causing abnormal fibrillin.

· Scurvy - caused by a dietary deficiency in vitamin C, leading to abnormal collagen.

· Ehlers-Danlos syndrome - deficient type III collagen- a genetic disease causing progressive deterioration of collagens, with different EDS types affecting different sites in the body, such as joints, heart valves, organ walls, arterial walls, etc.

· Loeys-Dietz syndrome - a genetic disease related to Marfan syndrome, with an emphasis on vascular deterioration.

· Pseudoxanthoma elasticum - an autosomal recessive hereditary disease, caused by calcification and fragmentation of elastic fibres, affecting the skin, the eyes and the cardiovascular system.

· Systemic lupus erythematosus - a chronic, multisystem, inflammatory disorder of probable autoimmune etiology, occurring predominantly in young women.

· Osteogenesis imperfecta (brittle bone disease) - caused by insufficient production of good quality collagen to produce healthy, strong bones.

· Fibrodysplasia ossificans progressiva - disease of the Connective tissue, caused by a defective gene which turns Connective tissue into bone.

· Spontaneous pneumothorax - collapsed lung, believed to be related to subtle abnormalities in Connective tissue.

· Sarcoma - a neoplastic process originating within Connective tissue.

Pelvic inflammatory disease

Pelvic inflammatory disease (or disorder) is a generic term for inflammation of the female uterus, fallopian tubes, and/or ovaries as it progresses to scar formation with adhesions to nearby tissues and organs. This may lead to tissue necrosis and sometimes abscess formation whereby pus can be released into the peritoneum. Pelvic inflammatory disease is often associated with sexually transmitted infections, as it is a common result of such infections.

Intervention

An intervention is an orchestrated attempt by one, or often many, people (usually family and friends) to get someone to seek professional help with an addiction or some kind of traumatic event or crisis, or other serious problem. The term intervention is most often used when the traumatic event involves addiction to drugs or other items. intervention can also refer to the act of using a technique within a therapy session.

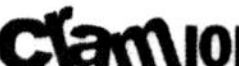

Fluticasone

Fluticasone is a synthetic glucocorticoid.
Both the furoate and propionate forms are used as topical anti-inflammatories:

· Fluticasone propionate

· Fluticasone furoate .

Vasoconstriction

Vasoconstriction is the narrowing of the blood vessels resulting from contraction of the muscular wall of the vessels, particularly the large arteries, small arterioles and veins. The process is the opposite of vasodilation, the widening of blood vessels. The process is particularly important in staunching hemorrhage and acute blood loss.

Rhinovirus

Human Rhinovirus A

Human Rhinovirus B

Human Rhinovirus C
Rhinovirus was a genus of the Picornaviridae family of viruses. It has been now merged into Enteroviruses, a group of Picornaviridae that includes Poliovirus, Coxsackie A virus, and Hepatitis A.

Rhinoviruses are the most common viral infective agents in humans, and a causative agent of the common cold. It is lytic in nature.

Pathophysiology

Pathophysiology is the study of the changes of normal mechanical, physical, and biochemical functions, either caused by a disease, it is the branch of medicine which deals with any disturbances of body functions, caused by disease or prodromal symptoms.
An alternate definition is `the study of the biological and physical manifestations of disease as they correlate with the underlying abnormalities and physiological disturbances.`

The study of pathology and the study of Pathophysiology often involves substantial overlap in diseases and processes, but pathology emphasizes direct observations, while Pathophysiology emphasizes quantifiable measurements.

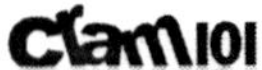

Hypoxia

Hypoxia, is a pathological condition in which the body as a whole (generalized hypoxia) or a region of the body (tissue hypoxia) is deprived of adequate oxygen supply. Variations in arterial oxygen concentrations can be part of the normal physiology, for example, during strenuous physical exercise. A mismatch between oxygen supply and its demand at the cellular level may result in a hypoxic condition.

Marche a petit pas

Marche à petits pas [mahrsh ah puh-TEE PAH] (`gait with little steps`) is a type of gait disorder characterised by an abnormal short stepped gait with upright stance (in strict sense, as opposed to generally stooping short-stepped gait of Parkinson`s disease), seen in various neurological (or ) disorders. It can be further differentiated from `Parkinsonian gait` by normal arm swing (as opposed to no arm swing in Parkinsonism). Some people refer to all forms of short-stepped gaits, including Parkinsonian gait, as Marche a petit pas in a loose sense.

Collagen

Collagen is a group of naturally occurring proteins. In nature, it is found exclusively in animals. It is the main protein of connective tissue.

Keratinocyte

Keratinocytes are the predominant cell type in the epidermis, the outermost layer of the human skin, constituting 95% of the cells found there. Those keratinocytes found in the basal layer (Stratum germinativum) of the skin are sometimes referred to as "basal cells" or "basal keratinocytes". The primary function of keratinocytes is the formation of a barrier against environmental damage such as pathogens (bacteria, fungi, parasites, viruses) heat, UV radiation and water loss.

Hurler syndrome

Hurler syndrome, also known as mucopolysaccharidosis type I (MPS I), Hurler`s disease or gargoylism, is a genetic disorder that results in the buildup of mucopolysaccharides due to a deficiency of alpha-L iduronidase, an enzyme responsible for the degradation of mucopolysaccharides in lysosomes.[:544] Without this enzyme, a buildup of heparan sulfate and dermatan sulfate occurs in the body. Symptoms appear during childhood and early death can occur due to organ damage.

MPS I is divided into three subtypes based on severity of symptoms.

Omalizumab

Omalizumab (Xolair, Genentech / Novartis) is a humanized antibody drug approved for patients with moderate-to-severe or severe allergic asthma, which is caused by hypersensitivity reactions to certain harmless environmental substances. Omalizumab`s cost is high ($10,000 to $30,000 per year), as compared to other drugs used for asthma, and hence Omalizumab is mainly prescribed for patients with severe, persistent asthma, which cannot be controlled even with high doses of corticosteroids. Like other protein and antibody drugs, Omalizumab causes anaphylaxis (a life-threatening systemic allergic reaction) in 1 to 2 patients per 1,000.

Pseudoxanthoma elasticum	Pseudoxanthoma elasticum is a genetic disease that causes fragmentation and mineralization of elastic fibers in some tissues. The most common problems arise in the skin and eyes, and later in blood vessels in the form of premature atherosclerosis. PXE is caused by autosomal recessive mutations in the ABCC6 gene on the short arm of chromosome 16 (16p13.1).
Bronchioles	The Bronchioles or bronchioli are the first airway branches that no longer contain cartilage. They are branches of the bronchi. The Bronchioles terminate by entering the circular sacs called alveoli.

Chapter 4. Inflammatory Mediators and Pathways

Asthma	Asthma is characterized by a predisposition to chronic inflammation of the lungs in which the airways (bronchi) are reversibly narrowed. Asthma affects 7% of the population of the United States, 6.5% of British people and a total of 300 million worldwide. During Asthma attacks (exacerbations of Asthma), the smooth muscle cells in the bronchi constrict, the airways become inflamed and swollen, and breathing becomes difficult.
Leukocytes	White blood cells are cells of the immune system defending the body against both infectious disease and foreign materials. Five different and diverse types of Leukocytes exist, but they are all produced and derived from a multipotent cell in the bone marrow known as a hematopoietic stem cell. Leukocytes are found throughout the body, including the blood and lymphatic system.
Factor XII	Hageman factor is a plasma protein , an enzyme (EC 3.4.21.38) of the serine protease (or serine endopeptidase) class. In humans, Factor XII is encoded by the F12 gene. It is part of the coagulation cascade and activates factor XI and prekallikrein.
Metabolism	Metabolism is the set of chemical reactions that happen in living organisms to maintain life. These processes allow organisms to grow and reproduce, maintain their structures, and respond to their environments. Metabolism is usually divided into two categories.
Prostaglandin	A Prostaglandin is any member of a group of lipid compounds that are derived enzymatically from fatty acids and have important functions in the animal body. Every Prostaglandin contains 20 carbon atoms, including a 5-carbon ring. They are mediators and have a variety of strong physiological effects, such as regulating the contraction and relaxation of smooth muscle tissue.
Protein	Proteins are organic compounds made of amino acids arranged in a linear chain and folded into a globular form. The amino acids in a polymer chain are joined together by the peptide bonds between the carboxyl and amino groups of adjacent amino acid residues. The sequence of amino acids in a protein is defined by the sequence of a gene, which is encoded in the genetic code.
Growth factor	A Growth factor is a naturally occurring substance capable of stimulating cellular growth, proliferation and cellular differentiation. Usually it is a protein or a steroid hormone. Growth factors are important for regulating a variety of cellular processes.
Neuroendocrine	Neuroendocrine [IPA nÊŠÉ™roÊŠËˆÉ›ndÉ™krÉªn] cells are cells that release a hormone into the circulating blood in response to a neural stimulus. These hormones may be amines, neuropeptides, or specialized amino acids. They package the hormones in vesicles and send these packages via long processes to blood vessels.

Pathology

Pathology is the study and diagnosis of disease through examination of organs, tissues, bodily fluids, and whole bodies (autopsies). The term also encompasses the related scientific study of disease processes, called General Pathology.
Medical Pathology is divided in two main branches, Anatomical Pathology and Clinical Pathology.

Omalizumab

Omalizumab (Xolair, Genentech / Novartis) is a humanized antibody drug approved for patients with moderate-to-severe or severe allergic asthma, which is caused by hypersensitivity reactions to certain harmless environmental substances. Omalizumab`s cost is high ($10,000 to $30,000 per year), as compared to other drugs used for asthma, and hence Omalizumab is mainly prescribed for patients with severe, persistent asthma, which cannot be controlled even with high doses of corticosteroids. Like other protein and antibody drugs, Omalizumab causes anaphylaxis (a life-threatening systemic allergic reaction) in 1 to 2 patients per 1,000.

Syndrome

In medicine and psychology, the term syndrome refers to the association of several clinically recognizable features, signs (observed by a physician), symptoms (reported by the patient), phenomena or characteristics that often occur together, so that the presence of one feature alerts the physician to the presence of the others. In recent decades the term has been used outside of medicine to refer to a combination of phenomena seen in association.
The term syndrome derives from its Greek roots and means literally `run together`, as the features do.

Multiple inert gas elimination technique

Multiple inert gas elimination technique is a technique used mainly in pneumology, that involves measuring mixed venous, arterial, and mixed expired concentrations of six infused inert gases, shows a shunt, dead space, and the general ventilation versus blood flow (Va/Q).
It is a good technique for establishing emphysema or chronic bronchitis.

`.

Allergen

An Allergen is a nonparasitic antigen capable of stimulating a type-I hypersensitivity reaction in atopic individuals.
Most humans mount significant Immunoglobulin E responses only as a defense against parasitic infections. However, some individuals mount an IgE response against common environmental antigens.

Signal

In physiology, a signal is an electric quantity (voltage or current or field strength), caused by chemical reactions of charged ions. Another use of the term lies in describing the transfer of information between and within cells, as in signal transduction.

Chapter 4. Inflammatory Mediators and Pathways

Bronchoalveolar lavage	Bronchoalveolar lavage (BAL) is a medical procedure in which a bronchoscope is passed through the mouth or nose into the lungs and fluid is squirted into a small part of the lung and then recollected for examination. BAL is typically performed to diagnose lung disease. In particular, BAL is commonly used to diagnose infections in people with immune system problems, pneumonia in people on ventilators, some types of lung cancer, and scarring of the lung (interstitial lung disease).
Calcium channel	A Calcium channel is an ion channel which displays selective permeabiltiy to calcium ions. It is sometimes synonymous as voltage-dependent calcium channel, although there are also ligand-gated calcium channels. Comparison tables The following tables explain gating, gene, location and function of different types of calcium channels, both voltage and ligand-gated.
Macrophages	Macrophages are white blood cells within tissues, produced by the division of monocytes. Human Macrophages are about 21 micrometres (0.00083 in) in diameter. Monocytes and Macrophages are phagocytes, acting in both non-specific defense (innate immunity) as well as to help initiate specific defense mechanisms (adaptive immunity) of vertebrate animals.
Lung	The Lung or pulmonary system is the essential respiration organ in all air-breathing animals, including most tetrapods, a few fish and a few snails. In mammals and the more complex life forms, the two Lungs are located in the chest on either side of the heart. Their principal function is to transport oxygen from the atmosphere into the bloodstream, and to release carbon dioxide from the bloodstream into the atmosphere.
Intervention	An intervention is an orchestrated attempt by one, or often many, people (usually family and friends) to get someone to seek professional help with an addiction or some kind of traumatic event or crisis, or other serious problem. The term intervention is most often used when the traumatic event involves addiction to drugs or other items. intervention can also refer to the act of using a technique within a therapy session.
Mycoplasma pneumonia	Mycoplasma pneumonia is a form of bacterial pneumonia which is caused by the bacteria species Mycoplasma pneumoniae. Disease from mycoplasma is usually mild to moderate in severity. The symptoms are usually mild enough that the patient may remain ambulatory throughout the illness.

Surfactant	Surfactants are wetting agents that lower the surface tension of a liquid, allowing easier spreading, and lower the interfacial tension between two liquids. The term Surfactant is a blend of surface active agent. Surfactants are usually organic compounds that are amphiphilic, meaning they contain both hydrophobic groups (their `tails`) and hydrophilic groups (their `heads`).
Curcumin	Curcumin is the principal Curcuminoid of the popular Indian spice turmeric, which is a member of the ginger family (Zingiberaceae). The other two Curcuminoids are desmethoxyCurcumin and bis-desmethoxyCurcumin. The Curcuminoids are polyphenols and are responsible for the yellow color of turmeric.
Cystic fibrosis	Cystic fibrosis (also known as Cystic fibrosis, mucovoidosis,) is a genetic disorder known to be an inherited disease of the secretory glands, including the glands that make mucus and sweat. The hallmarks of Cystic fibrosis are salty tasting skin, normal appetite but poor growth and poor weight gain, excess mucus production, frequent chest infections and coughing/shortness of breath. Males can be infertile due to the condition Congenital absence of the vas deferens.
Duffy antigen	The Duffy antigen is a protein located on the surface of red blood cells and is named after the patient in which it was discovered. In humans, this protein is encoded by the Duffy antigenRC gene. The protein encoded by this gene is a glycosylated membrane protein and a non-specific receptor for several chemokines.
Defensins	Defensins are small cysteine-rich cationic proteins found in both vertebrates and invertebrates. They are active against bacteria, fungi and many enveloped and nonenveloped viruses. They consist of 18-45 amino acids including six (in vertebrates) to 8 conserved cysteine residues.
Dendritic cell	Dendritic cells are immune cells that form part of the mammalian immune system. Their main function is to process antigen material and present it on the surface to other cells of the immune system, thus functioning as antigen-presenting cells. They act as messengers between the innate and adaptive immunity. Dendritic cells are present in small quantities in tissues that are in contact with the external environment, mainly the skin (where there is a specialized Dendritic cell type called Langerhans cells) and the inner lining of the nose, lungs, stomach and intestines. They can also be found in an immature state in the blood.

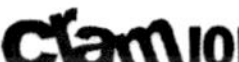

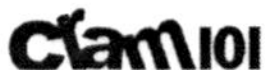

Disease	A disease or medical condition is an abnormal condition of an organism that impairs bodily functions, associated with specific symptoms and signs. It may be caused by external factors, such as invading organisms, or it may be caused by internal dysfunctions, such as autoimmune diseases. In human beings, `disease` is often used more broadly to refer to any condition that causes pain, dysfunction, distress, social problems, and/or death to the person afflicted, or similar problems for those in contact with the person.
Fibroblast	A Fibroblast is a type of cell that synthesizes the extracellular matrix and collagen, the structural framework (stroma) for animal tissues, and plays a critical role in wound healing. Fibroblasts are the most common cells of connective tissue in animals. Fibroblasts and fibrocytes are two states of the same cells, the former being the activated state, the latter the less active state, concerned with maintenance.
Mast cell	A Mast cell is a resident cell of several types of tissues and contains many granules rich in histamine and heparin. Although best known for their role in allergy and anaphylaxis, Mast cells play an important protective role as well, being intimately involved in wound healing and defense against pathogens. Mast cells were first described by Paul Ehrlich in his 1878 doctoral thesis on the basis of their unique staining characteristics and large granules.
Hurler syndrome	Hurler syndrome, also known as mucopolysaccharidosis type I (MPS I), Hurler`s disease or gargoylism, is a genetic disorder that results in the buildup of mucopolysaccharides due to a deficiency of alpha-L iduronidase, an enzyme responsible for the degradation of mucopolysaccharides in lysosomes.[:544] Without this enzyme, a buildup of heparan sulfate and dermatan sulfate occurs in the body. Symptoms appear during childhood and early death can occur due to organ damage. MPS I is divided into three subtypes based on severity of symptoms.
Inflammation	Inflammation is the complex biological response of vascular tissues to harmful stimuli, such as pathogens, damaged cells, or irritants. Inflammation is a protective attempt by the organism to remove the injurious stimuli as well as initiate the healing process for the tissue. Inflammation is not a synonym for infection.

Antigen presentation	Antigen presentation is a process in the body's immune system by which macrophages, dendritic cells and other cell types capture antigens and then enable their recognition by T-cells. The basis of adaptive immunity lies in the capacity of immune cells to distinguish between the body's own cells, and infectious pathogens. The host's cells express 'self' antigens that identify them as such.
Interferon	Interferons (IFNs) are proteins made and released by lymphocytes in response to the presence of pathogens--such as viruses, bacteria, or parasites--or tumor cells. They allow communication between cells to trigger the protective defenses of the immune system that eradicate pathogens or tumors. Interferons belong to the large class of glycoproteins known as cytokines.
Interleukins	Interleukins are a group of cytokines (secreted proteins/signaling molecules) that were first seen to be expressed by white blood cells (leukocytes), The term interleukine, (inter-) as a means of communication, (-leukin) deriving from the fact that many of these proteins are produced by leukocytes and act on leukocytes. The name is something of a relic though (the term was coined by Dr. Paetkau, University of Victoria); it has since been found that Interleukins are produced by a wide variety of body cells. The function of the immune system depends in a large part on Interleukins, and rare deficiencies of a number of them have been described, all featuring autoimmune diseases or immune deficiency.
Necrosis	Necrosis is the premature death of cells and living tissue. Necrosis is caused by factors external to the cell or tissue, such as infection, toxins, or trauma. This is in contrast to apoptosis, which is a naturally occurring cause of cellular death.
Colony-stimulating factor	Colony-stimulating factors are secreted glycoproteins which bind to receptor proteins on the surfaces of hemopoietic stem cells and thereby activate intracellular signaling pathways which can cause the cells to proliferate and differentiate into a specific kind of blood cell . They may be synthesized and administered exogenously. However, such molecules can at a latter stage be detected, since they differ slightly from the endogenous ones in e.g.

Granulocyte-macrophage colony-stimulating factor	Granulocyte-macrophage colony-stimulating factor, often abbreviated to GM-CSF, is a protein secreted by macrophages, T cells, mast cells, endothelial cells and fibroblasts. GM-CSF is a cytokine that functions as a white blood cell growth factor. GM-CSF stimulates stem cells to produce granulocytes and monocytes.
Hyperplasia	Hyperplasia (or `hypergenesis`) is a general term referring to the proliferation of cells within an organ or tissue beyond that which is ordinarily seen (e.g. constantly dividing cells). Hyperplasia may result in the gross enlargement of an organ, the formation of a benign tumor, or may be visible only under a microscope. Hyperplasia is different from hypertrophy in that the adaptive cell change in hypertrophy is by increased cellular size only, whereas in Hyperplasia it is by increased cellular number.
Protease	This article discusses primarily the structure and properties of proteolytic enzymes. For medical, surgical and related applications of several Proteases, see article: Proteases (medical and related uses) Proteases break down proteins. A Protease is any enzyme that conducts proteolysis, that is, begins protein catabolism by hydrolysis of the peptide bonds that link amino acids together in the polypeptide chain, which form a molecule of protein.
Erythromycin	Erythromycin is a macrolide antibiotic that has an antimicrobial spectrum similar to or slightly wider than that of penicillin, and is often used for people who have an allergy to penicillins. For respiratory tract infections, it has better coverage of atypical organisms, including mycoplasma and Legionellosis. It was first marketed by Eli Lilly and Company, and it is today commonly known as EES (Erythromycin ethylsuccinate, an ester prodrug that is commonly administered).
Colitis	Colitis is a chronic digestive disease characterized by inflammation of the colon. Colitis is one of a group of conditions which are inflammatory and auto-immune, affecting the tissue that lines the gastrointestinal system (the large and small intestine). It is classed as an inflammatory bowel disease (IBD), not to be confused with irritable bowel syndrome (IBS).
Ulcerative colitis	Ulcerative colitis (Colitis ulcerosa, Ulcerative colitis) is a form of inflammatory bowel disease (IBD). Ulcerative colitis is a form of colitis, a disease of the intestine, specifically the large intestine or colon, that includes characteristic ulcers, or open sores, in the colon. The main symptom of active disease is usually constant diarrhea mixed with blood, of gradual onset.
Usual interstitial pneumonia	Usual interstitial pneumonia, commonly abbreviated Usual interstitial pneumonia, is the name of a histopathological pattern seen in diffuse lung diseases, i.e. interstitial lung diseases. It is classified as an idiopathic interstitial pneumonia, and may be idiopathic, i.e. the cause is unknown, or due to a known cause, e.g. asbestos exposure.

	The hallmarks of Usual interstitial pneumonia are interstitial inflammation, i.e. inflammation of the alveolar walls, and fibrosis (scarring).
Vascular endothelial growth factor	Vascular endothelial growth factor is a signal protein produced by cells that stimulates the growth of new blood vessels. It is part of the system that restores the oxygen supply to tissues when blood circulation is inadequate. Vascular endothelial growth factor's normal function is to create new blood vessels during embryonic development, new blood vessels after injury, muscle following exercise, and new vessels (collateral circulation) to bypass blocked vessels.
Ehlers-Danlos syndrome	Ehlers-Danlos syndrome is a group of inherited connective tissue disorders, caused by a defect in the synthesis of collagen (a protein in connective tissue). The collagen in connective tissue helps tissues to resist deformation (decreases its elasticity). In the skin, muscles, ligaments, blood vessels, and visceral organs collagen plays a very significant role and with increased elasticity, secondary to abnormal collagen, pathology results.
Azurophil	Azurophil is the term used to refer to objects that are readily staining with an azure dye. The term is used especially in reference to certain cytoplasmic granules in white blood cells, particularly hyperchromatin and reddish purple granules of certain blood cells. As another example, neutrophils carry an arsenal of anti-microbial defensins within their Azurophils, which eventually fuse with phagocytic vacuoles.
Matrix	The hair matrix produces the actual hair shaft as well as the inner and outer root sheaths.
Matrix metalloproteinases	Matrix metalloproteinases are zinc-dependent endopeptidases; other family members are adamalysins, serralysins, and astacins. The MMPs belong to a larger family of proteases known as the metzincin superfamily. Collectively they are capable of degrading all kinds of extracellular matrix proteins, but also can process a number of bioactive molecules.

Glucocorticoid	Glucocorticoids are a class of steroid hormones that bind to the Glucocorticoid receptor (GR), which is present in almost every vertebrate animal cell. The name Glucocorticoid derives from their role in the regulation of the metabolism of glucose, their synthesis in the adrenal cortex, and their steroidal structure . GCs are part of the feedback mechanism in the immune system that turns immune activity (inflammation) down.
Cathepsin	Cathepsins are proteases: proteins that break apart other proteins, found in many types of cells including those in all animals. There are approximately a dozen members of this family, which are distinguished by their structure, catalytic mechanism, and which proteins they cleave. Most of the members become activated at the low pH found in lysosomes.
Cystatin C	Cystatin C or cystatin 3 (formerly gamma trace, post-gamma-globulin or neuroendocrine basic polypeptide), a protein encoded by the CST3 gene, is mainly used as a biomarker of kidney function. Recently, it has been studied for its role in predicting new-onset or deteriorating cardiovascular disease. It also seems to play a role in brain disorders involving amyloid (a specific type of protein deposition), such as Alzheimer`s disease.
Obstructive lung disease	Obstructive lung disease is a category of respiratory disease characterized by airway obstruction. MeSH includes the following in this category: · Asthma · Bronchitis · Chronic obstructive pulmonary disease Cystic fibrosis is sometimes also included in this category. FEV1/FVC ratio is usually decreased.

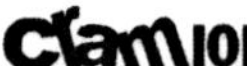

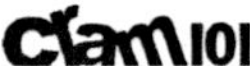

Emphysema	Emphysema is a lung disease, characterized by an abnormal, permanent enlargement of air spaces distal to the terminal bronchioles. The disease is coupled with the destruction of walls, but without obvious fibrosis. It is often caused by exposure to toxic chemicals, including long-term exposure to tobacco smoke.
Deficiency	A deficiency is a lack of something... Example : there is a deficiency of oxygen in the air. · In mathematics, a deficient number is a number n for which $\sigma(n) < 2n$.
Bleomycin	Bleomycin is a glycopeptide antibiotic produced by the bacterium Streptomyces verticillus. Bleomycin refers to a family of structurally related compounds. When used as an anticancer agent, the chemotherapeutical forms are primarily bleomycin A_2 and B_2.
Plasmin	Plasmin is an important enzyme present in blood that degrades many blood plasma proteins, most notably, fibrin clots. The degradation of fibrin is termed fibrinolysis. In humans, the Plasmin protein is encoded by the PLG gene.
Granulocytes	Granulocytes are a category of white blood cells characterised by the presence of granules in their cytoplasm. They are also called polymorphonuclear leukocytes (PMN or PML) because of the varying shapes of the nucleus, which is usually lobed into three segments. In common parlance, the term polymorphonuclear leukocyte often refers specifically to neutrophil Granulocytes, the most abundant of the Granulocytes.
Bronchoscopy	Bronchoscopy is a technique of visualizing the inside of the airways for diagnostic and therapeutic purposes. An instrument (bronchoscope) is inserted into the airways, usually through the nose or mouth, or occasionally through a tracheostomy. This allows the practitioner to examine the patient's airways for abnormalities such as foreign bodies, bleeding, tumors, or inflammation.
Insulin-like growth factors	The Insulin-like growth factors (Insulin-like growth factorss) are polypeptides with high sequence similarity to insulin. Insulin-like growth factorss are part of a complex system that cells use to communicate with their physiologic environment. This complex system (often referred to as the Insulin-like growth factors \`axis\`) consists of two cell-surface receptors (Insulin-like growth factors1R and Insulin-like growth factors2R), two ligands (Insulin-like growth factors-1 and Insulin-like growth factors-2), a family of six high-affinity Insulin-like growth factors binding proteins (Insulin-like growth factorsBP 1-6), as well as associated Insulin-like growth factorsBP degrading enzymes, referred to collectively as proteases.

Keratinocyte	Keratinocytes are the predominant cell type in the epidermis, the outermost layer of the human skin, constituting 95% of the cells found there. Those keratinocytes found in the basal layer (Stratum germinativum) of the skin are sometimes referred to as "basal cells" or "basal keratinocytes". The primary function of keratinocytes is the formation of a barrier against environmental damage such as pathogens (bacteria, fungi, parasites, viruses) heat, UV radiation and water loss.
Connective tissue	Connective tissue is a form of fibrous tissue. It is one of the four types of tissue in traditional classifications (the others being epithelial, muscle, and nervous tissue). Collagen is the main protein of Connective tissue in animals and the most abundant protein in mammals, making up about 25% of the total protein content. Fiber types as follows: · collagenous fibers · elastic fibers · Bone Marrow Various Connective tissue conditions have been identified; these can be both inherited and environmental. · Marfan syndrome - a genetic disease causing abnormal fibrillin. · Scurvy - caused by a dietary deficiency in vitamin C, leading to abnormal collagen. · Ehlers-Danlos syndrome - deficient type III collagen- a genetic disease causing progressive deterioration of collagens, with different EDS types affecting different sites in the body, such as joints, heart valves, organ walls, arterial walls, etc. · Loeys-Dietz syndrome - a genetic disease related to Marfan syndrome, with an emphasis on vascular deterioration.

· Pseudoxanthoma elasticum - an autosomal recessive hereditary disease, caused by calcification and fragmentation of elastic fibres, affecting the skin, the eyes and the cardiovascular system.

· Systemic lupus erythematosus - a chronic, multisystem, inflammatory disorder of probable autoimmune etiology, occurring predominantly in young women.

· Osteogenesis imperfecta (brittle bone disease) - caused by insufficient production of good quality collagen to produce healthy, strong bones.

· Fibrodysplasia ossificans progressiva - disease of the Connective tissue, caused by a defective gene which turns Connective tissue into bone.

· Spontaneous pneumothorax - collapsed lung, believed to be related to subtle abnormalities in Connective tissue.

· Sarcoma - a neoplastic process originating within Connective tissue.

Constipation

Constipation, costiveness,) experiences hard feces (faeces) that are difficult to expel. This usually happens because the colon absorbs too much water from the food. If the food moves through the gastro-intestinal tract too slowly, the colon may absorb too much water, resulting in feces that are dry and hard.

Epithelial-mesenchymal transition

Epithelial-mesenchymal transition is a hypothesized program of development of biological cells characterized by loss of cell adhesion, repression of E-cadherin expression, and increased cell mobility. Epithelial mesenchymal transition may be essential for numerous developmental processes including mesoderm formation and neural tube formation.

Induction

Several oncogenic pathways (peptide growth factors, Src, Ras, Ets, integrin, Wnt/beta-catenin and Notch) may induce Epithelial mesenchymal transition. In particular, Ras-MAPK has been shown to activate two related transcription factors known as Snail and Slug.

Volume	The Volume of any solid, liquid, gas, plasma, or vacuum is how much three-dimensional space it occupies, often quantified numerically. One-dimensional figures (such as lines) and two-dimensional shapes (such as squares) are assigned zero Volume in the three-dimensional space. Volume is commonly presented in units such as cubic meters, cubic centimeters, liters, or milliliters.
Platelet	Platelets, or thrombocytes , are small, irregularly-shaped anuclear cells , 2-3 Âµm in diameter, which are derived from fragmentation of precursor megakaryocytes. The average lifespan of a Platelet is between 8 and 12 days. Platelets play a fundamental role in hemostasis and are a natural source of growth factors.
Diagnosis	In medicine, diagnosis (plural, diagnoses) is the process of identifying a medical condition or disease by its signs, symptoms, and from the results of various diagnostic procedures. The conclusion reached through this process is called a diagnosis. The term \`diagnostic criteria\` designates the combination of signs, symptoms, and test results that allows the health care practitioner to ascertain the diagnosis of the respective disease.
Budesonide	Budesonide is a glucocorticoid steroid for the treatment of asthma, non-infectious rhinitis (including hay fever and other allergies), and for treatment and prevention of nasal polyposis. Additionally, it is used for Crohn's disease (inflammatory bowel disease). It is marketed by AstraZeneca as a nasal inhalant under the brand name Rhinocort (in Denmark, as Rhinosol), as an oral inhalant under the brand name Pulmicort, and as either an enema or a modified release oral capsule under the brand name Entocort.
Corticosteroid	Corticosteroids are a class of steroid hormones that are produced in the adrenal cortex. Corticosteroids are involved in a wide range of physiologic systems such as stress response, immune response and regulation of inflammation, carbohydrate metabolism, protein catabolism, blood electrolyte levels, and behavior. · Glucocorticoids such as cortisol control carbohydrate, fat and protein metabolism and are anti-inflammatory by preventing phospholipid release, decreasing eosinophil action and a number of other mechanisms. · Mineralocorticoids such as aldosterone control electrolyte and water levels, mainly by promoting sodium retention in the kidney.

Some common natural hormones are corticosterone ($C_{21}H_{30}O_4$), cortisone ($C_{21}H_{28}O_5$, 17-hydroxy-11-dehydrocorticosterone) and aldosterone.

Dose

A dose is a quantity of something (chemical, physical, or biological) that may impact an organism biologically; the greater the quantity, the larger the dose. In nutrition, the term is usually applied to how much of a specific nutrient is in a person's diet or in a particular food, meal, or dietary supplement. In medicine, the term is usually applied to the quantity of a drug or other agent administered for therapeutic purposes.

Monitoring

To monitor or Monitoring generally means to be aware of the state of a system. Below are specific examples:

· to observe a situation for any changes which may occur over time, using a monitor or measuring device of some sort:

· Baby monitor, medical monitor, Heart rate monitor

· BioMonitoring

· Cure Monitoring for composite materials manufacturing

· Deformation Monitoring

· Election Monitoring

· Mining Monitoring

· Natural hazard Monitoring

· Network Monitoring

· Structural Monitoring

· Website Monitoring

· Futures Monitoring, Media Monitoring service

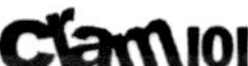

	· to observe the behaviour or communications of individuals or groups · Monitoring competence at a task. · Clinical Monitoring for new medical drugs Monitoring Integration Platform · Indiktor - Monitoring Integration Platform .
Chronic obstructive pulmonary disease	Chronic obstructive pulmonary disease refers to chronic bronchitis and emphysema, a pair of two commonly co-existing diseases of the lungs in which the airways become narrowed. This leads to a limitation of the flow of air to and from the lungs causing shortness of breath. In contrast to asthma, the limitation of airflow is poorly reversible and usually gets progressively worse over time.
Epidemic	In epidemiology, an Epidemic occurs when new cases of a certain disease, in a given human population, and during a given period, substantially exceed what is `expected,` based on recent experience . (An epizootic is the analogous circumstance within an animal population). In recent usages, the disease is not required to be communicable; examples include cancer or heart disease.
Cell type	A Cell type is a distinct morphological or functional form of cell. When a cell switches state from one Cell type to another, it undergoes cellular differentiation. A complete list of distinct Cell types in the adult human body may include about 210 distinct types.
Afferent neurons	In the nervous system, afferent neurons (otherwise known as sensory or receptor neurons), carry nerve impulses from receptors or sense organs toward the central nervous system. This term can also be used to describe relative connections between structures. afferent neurons communicate with specialized interneurons.

Artery	The arterial system is the higher-pressure portion of the circulatory system. Arterial pressure varies between the peak pressure during heart contraction, called the systolic pressure, and the minimum, or diastolic pressure between contractions, when the heart expands and refills. This pressure variation within the Artery produces the pulse which is observable in any Artery, and reflects heart activity.
Paracetamol	Paracetamol or acetaminophen) is a widely used over-the-counter analgesic (pain reliever) and antipyretic (fever reducer). However, its effectiveness alone as an antipyretic has been questioned. It is commonly used for the relief of headaches, and other minor aches and pains, and is a major ingredient in numerous cold and flu remedies.
Coronary artery disease	(Coronary artery disease or atherosclerotic heart disease) is the end result of the accumulation of atheromatous plaques within the walls of the coronary arteries that supply the myocardium (the muscle of the heart) with oxygen and nutrients. It is sometimes also called coronary heart disease (CHD), although Coronary artery disease is the most common cause of CHD, it is not the only one. Coronary artery disease is the leading cause of death worldwide.
Inhalant	Inhalants are a broad range of drugs in the forms of gases, aerosols, including organic solvents (found in cleaning products, fast-drying glues, and nail polish removers), fuels (gasoline (petrol) and kerosene) and propellant gases such as freon and compressed hydrofluorocarbons that are used in aerosol cans such as hairspray, whipped cream and non-stick cooking spray.
Neurotransmitter	Neurotransmitters are endogenous chemicals which relay, amplify, and modulate signals between a neuron and another cell. Neurotransmitters are packaged into synaptic vesicles that cluster beneath the membrane on the presynaptic side of a synapse, and are released into the synaptic cleft, where they bind to receptors in the membrane on the postsynaptic side of the synapse. Release of Neurotransmitters usually follows arrival of an action potential at the synapse, but may follow graded electrical potentials.
Atropine	Atropine is a tropane alkaloid extracted from deadly nightshade (Atropa belladonna), jimsonweed (Datura stramonium), mandrake (Mandragora officinarum) and other plants of the family Solanaceae. It is a secondary metabolite of these plants and serves as a drug with a wide variety of effects. It is a competitive antagonist for the muscarinic acetylcholine receptor.

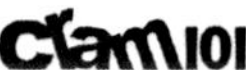

Chapter 4. Inflammatory Mediators and Pathways

Axon

An Axon or nerve fiber is a long, slender projection of a nerve cell, that conducts electrical impulses away from the neuron's cell body or soma.
An Axon is one of two types of protoplasmic protrusions that extrude from the cell body of a neuron, the other type being dendrites. Axons are distinguished from dendrites by several features, including shape (dendrites often taper while Axons usually maintain a constant radius), length (dendrites are restricted to a small region around the cell body while Axons can be much longer), and function (dendrites usually receive signals while Axons usually transmit them).

Catecholamines

Catecholamines are sympathomimetic 'fight-or-flight' hormones that are released by the adrenal glands in response to stress. They are part of the sympathetic nervous system.

They are called Catecholamines because they contain a catechol group, and are derived from the amino acid tyrosine.

Epinephrine

Epinephrine is a hormone and neurotransmitter. When produced in the body it increases heart rate, contracts blood vessels and dilates air passages and participates in the 'fight or flight' response of the sympathetic nervous system. It is a catecholamine, a sympathomimetic monoamine produced only by the adrenal glands from the amino acids phenylalanine and tyrosine.

Hormone

A Hormone is a chemical released by one or more cells that affects cells in other parts of the organism. Only a small amount of Hormone is required to alter cell metabolism. It is essentially a chemical messenger that transports a signal from one cell to another.

Atherosclerosis

Atherosclerosis is a condition in which an artery wall thickens as the result of a build-up of fatty materials such as cholesterol. It is a syndrome affecting arterial blood vessels, a chronic inflammatory response in the walls of arteries, in large part due to the accumulation of macrophage white blood cells and promoted by low-density lipoproteins (plasma proteins that carry cholesterol and triglycerides) without adequate removal of fats and cholesterol from the macrophages by functional high density lipoproteins (HDL), . It is commonly referred to as a hardening or furring of the arteries.

Angiotensin

Angiotensin, a protein, causes blood vessels to constrict, and drives blood pressure up. It is part of the renin-Angiotensin system, which is a major target for drugs that lower blood pressure. Angiotensin also stimulates the release of aldosterone from the adrenal cortex.

Bone

Bones are rigid organs that form part of the endoskeleton of vertebrates. They function to move, support, and protect the various organs of the body, produce red and white blood cells and store minerals. bone tissue is a type of dense connective tissue.

Brain natriuretic peptide

Brain natriuretic peptide now known as B-type natriuretic peptide (also Brain natriuretic peptide) or GC-B, is a 32 amino acid polypeptide secreted by the ventricles of the heart in response to excessive stretching of heart muscle cells (cardiomyocytes). Brain natriuretic peptide is named as such because it was originally identified in extracts of porcine brain, although in humans it is produced mainly in the cardiac ventricles.

Brain natriuretic peptide is co-secreted along with a 76 amino acid N-terminal fragment (NT-proBrain natriuretic peptide) which is biologically inactive.

Dopamine

Dopamine is a neurotransmitter that occurs in a wide variety of animals, including both vertebrates and invertebrates. In the brain, this phenethylamine functions as a neurotransmitter, activating the five types of Dopamine receptors--D_1, D_2, D_3, D_4, and D_5--and their variants. Dopamine is produced in several areas of the brain, including the substantia nigra and the ventral tegmental area.

Gas exchange

Gas exchange takes place at a respiratory surface--a boundary between the external environment and the interior of the organism. For unicellular organisms the respiratory surface is governed by Fick`s law, which determines that respiratory surfaces must have:

· a large surface area

· a thin permeable surface

· a moist exchange surface.

Many also have a mechanism to maximise the diffusion gradient by replenishing the source and/or sink.

	Control of respiration is due to rhythmical breathing generated by the phrenic nerve in order to stimulate contraction and relaxation of the diaphragm during inspiration and expiration.
Norepinephrine	Norepinephrine or noradrenaline (BAN) is a catecholamine with multiple roles including as a hormone and a neurotransmitter. As a stress hormone, Norepinephrine affects parts of the brain where attention and responding actions are controlled. Along with epinephrine, Norepinephrine also underlies the fight-or-flight response, directly increasing heart rate, triggering the release of glucose from energy stores, and increasing blood flow to skeletal muscle.
Renin-angiotensin system	The Renin-angiotensin system (RAS) or the renin-angiotensin-aldosterone system (RAAS) is a hormone system that regulates blood pressure and water (fluid) balance. When blood volume is low, the kidneys secrete renin. Renin stimulates the production of angiotensin.
Adrenomedullin	Adrenomedullin is a peptide associated with pheochromocytoma- a tumour arising from adrenal medulla. It was discovered in 1993. Adrenomedullin (AM) is a ubiquitously expressed peptide initially isolated from phaechromyctoma in 1993 (Kitamura et al., 1998).
Cortisol	Cortisol is a corticosteroid hormone or glucocorticoid produced by the adrenal cortex, that is part of the adrenal gland (in the zona fasciculata and the zona reticularis of the adrenal cortex). It is usually referred to as the \`stress hormone\` as it is involved in response to stress and anxiety, controlled by CRH. It increases blood pressure and blood sugar, and reduces immune responses. Various synthetic forms of Cortisol are used to treat a variety of different illnesses.
Estrogen	Estrogens (U.S., otherwise oEstrogens or Å“strogens) are a group of steroid compounds and functioning as the primary female sex hormone, their name comes from estrus/oistros (period of fertility for female mammals) + gen/gonos = to generate. Estrogens are used as part of some oral contraceptives, in Estrogen replacement therapy for postmenopausal women, and in hormone replacement therapy for transwomen. Like all steroid hormones, Estrogens readily diffuse across the cell membrane.

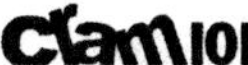

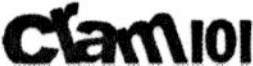

Glucagon	Glucagon is an important hormone involved in carbohydrate metabolism. Produced by the pancreas, it is released when blood glucose levels start to fall too low, causing the liver to convert stored glycogen into glucose and release it into the bloodstream, raising blood glucose levels and ultimately preventing the development of hypoglycemia. The action of Glucagon is thus opposite to that of insulin, which instructs the body`s cells to take in glucose from the blood.
Thyroid hormone	The Thyroid hormones, thyroxine (T_4) and triiodothyronine (T_3), are tyrosine-based hormones produced by the thyroid gland primarily responsible for regulation of metabolism. An important component in the synthesis of Thyroid hormones is iodine. The major form of Thyroid hormone in the blood is thyroxine (T_4), which has a longer half life than T_3.

Chapter 5. Pathogenic Mechanisms in Asthma and COPD

Marfan syndrome	Marfan syndrome is a genetic disorder of the connective tissue. It is sometimes inherited as a dominant trait. It is carried by a gene called FBN1, which encodes a connective protein called fibrillin-1. People have a pair of FBN1 genes.
Asthma	Asthma is characterized by a predisposition to chronic inflammation of the lungs in which the airways (bronchi) are reversibly narrowed. Asthma affects 7% of the population of the United States, 6.5% of British people and a total of 300 million worldwide. During Asthma attacks (exacerbations of Asthma), the smooth muscle cells in the bronchi constrict, the airways become inflamed and swollen, and breathing becomes difficult.
Bronchoalveolar lavage	Bronchoalveolar lavage (BAL) is a medical procedure in which a bronchoscope is passed through the mouth or nose into the lungs and fluid is squirted into a small part of the lung and then recollected for examination. BAL is typically performed to diagnose lung disease. In particular, BAL is commonly used to diagnose infections in people with immune system problems, pneumonia in people on ventilators, some types of lung cancer, and scarring of the lung (interstitial lung disease).
Bronchoscopy	Bronchoscopy is a technique of visualizing the inside of the airways for diagnostic and therapeutic purposes. An instrument (bronchoscope) is inserted into the airways, usually through the nose or mouth, or occasionally through a tracheostomy. This allows the practitioner to examine the patient's airways for abnormalities such as foreign bodies, bleeding, tumors, or inflammation.
Disease	A disease or medical condition is an abnormal condition of an organism that impairs bodily functions, associated with specific symptoms and signs. It may be caused by external factors, such as invading organisms, or it may be caused by internal dysfunctions, such as autoimmune diseases. In human beings, `disease` is often used more broadly to refer to any condition that causes pain, dysfunction, distress, social problems, and/or death to the person afflicted, or similar problems for those in contact with the person.
Factor XII	Hageman factor is a plasma protein , an enzyme (EC 3.4.21.38) of the serine protease (or serine endopeptidase) class. In humans, Factor XII is encoded by the F12 gene. It is part of the coagulation cascade and activates factor XI and prekallikrein.

Fibroblast

A Fibroblast is a type of cell that synthesizes the extracellular matrix and collagen, the structural framework (stroma) for animal tissues, and plays a critical role in wound healing. Fibroblasts are the most common cells of connective tissue in animals.

Fibroblasts and fibrocytes are two states of the same cells, the former being the activated state, the latter the less active state, concerned with maintenance.

Growth factor

A Growth factor is a naturally occurring substance capable of stimulating cellular growth, proliferation and cellular differentiation. Usually it is a protein or a steroid hormone. Growth factors are important for regulating a variety of cellular processes.

Lung

The Lung or pulmonary system is the essential respiration organ in all air-breathing animals, including most tetrapods, a few fish and a few snails. In mammals and the more complex life forms, the two Lungs are located in the chest on either side of the heart. Their principal function is to transport oxygen from the atmosphere into the bloodstream, and to release carbon dioxide from the bloodstream into the atmosphere.

Macrophages

Macrophages are white blood cells within tissues, produced by the division of monocytes. Human Macrophages are about 21 micrometres (0.00083 in) in diameter. Monocytes and Macrophages are phagocytes, acting in both non-specific defense (innate immunity) as well as to help initiate specific defense mechanisms (adaptive immunity) of vertebrate animals.

Mast cell

A Mast cell is a resident cell of several types of tissues and contains many granules rich in histamine and heparin. Although best known for their role in allergy and anaphylaxis, Mast cells play an important protective role as well, being intimately involved in wound healing and defense against pathogens.

Mast cells were first described by Paul Ehrlich in his 1878 doctoral thesis on the basis of their unique staining characteristics and large granules.

Pathology

Pathology is the study and diagnosis of disease through examination of organs, tissues, bodily fluids, and whole bodies (autopsies). The term also encompasses the related scientific study of disease processes, called General Pathology.
Medical Pathology is divided in two main branches, Anatomical Pathology and Clinical Pathology.

Pathophysiology

Pathophysiology is the study of the changes of normal mechanical, physical, and biochemical functions, either caused by a disease, it is the branch of medicine which deals with any disturbances of body functions, caused by disease or prodromal symptoms.

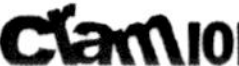

	An alternate definition is `the study of the biological and physical manifestations of disease as they correlate with the underlying abnormalities and physiological disturbances.` The study of pathology and the study of Pathophysiology often involves substantial overlap in diseases and processes, but pathology emphasizes direct observations, while Pathophysiology emphasizes quantifiable measurements.
Inflammation	Inflammation is the complex biological response of vascular tissues to harmful stimuli, such as pathogens, damaged cells, or irritants. Inflammation is a protective attempt by the organism to remove the injurious stimuli as well as initiate the healing process for the tissue. Inflammation is not a synonym for infection.
Bronchitis	Bronchitis is inflammation of the mucous membranes of the bronchi, the airways that carry airflow from the trachea into the lungs. Bronchitis can be classified into two categories, acute and chronic, each of which has unique etiologies, pathologies, and therapies. Acute Bronchitis is characterized by the development of a cough, with or without the production of sputum, mucus that is expectorated (coughed up) from the respiratory tract.
Defensins	Defensins are small cysteine-rich cationic proteins found in both vertebrates and invertebrates. They are active against bacteria, fungi and many enveloped and nonenveloped viruses. They consist of 18-45 amino acids including six (in vertebrates) to 8 conserved cysteine residues.
Dendritic cell	Dendritic cells are immune cells that form part of the mammalian immune system. Their main function is to process antigen material and present it on the surface to other cells of the immune system, thus functioning as antigen-presenting cells. They act as messengers between the innate and adaptive immunity. Dendritic cells are present in small quantities in tissues that are in contact with the external environment, mainly the skin (where there is a specialized Dendritic cell type called Langerhans cells) and the inner lining of the nose, lungs, stomach and intestines. They can also be found in an immature state in the blood.
Eosinophilic	Eosinophilic means loves eosin, and refers to the staining of certain tissues, cells, a dye. Eosin is an acidic dye; thus, the structure being stained is basic. Eosinophilic describes the appearance of cells and structures seen in histological sections that take up the staining dye eosin.

Chapter 5. Pathogenic Mechanisms in Asthma and COPD

Omalizumab	Omalizumab (Xolair, Genentech / Novartis) is a humanized antibody drug approved for patients with moderate-to-severe or severe allergic asthma, which is caused by hypersensitivity reactions to certain harmless environmental substances. Omalizumab`s cost is high ($10,000 to $30,000 per year), as compared to other drugs used for asthma, and hence Omalizumab is mainly prescribed for patients with severe, persistent asthma, which cannot be controlled even with high doses of corticosteroids. Like other protein and antibody drugs, Omalizumab causes anaphylaxis (a life-threatening systemic allergic reaction) in 1 to 2 patients per 1,000.
Group B Streptococcus	Infection with Group B Streptococcus can cause serious illness and , especially in newborn infants, the elderly, and patients with compromised immune systems. Group B streptococci are also prominent veterinary pathogens, because they can cause bovine mastitis (inflammation of the udder) in dairy cows. The species name `agalactiae` meaning `no milk`, alludes to this.
T cell	T cells or T lymphocytes belong to a group of white blood cells known as lymphocytes, and play a central role in cell-mediated immunity. They can be distinguished from other lymphocyte types, such as B cells and natural killer cells by the presence of a special receptor on their cell surface called T cell receptors (TCR). The abbreviation T, in T cell, stands for thymus, since this is the principal organ responsible for the T cell`s maturation.
Lymphocyte	A Lymphocyte is a type of white blood cell in the vertebrate immune system. Under the microscope, Lymphocytes can be divided into large granular Lymphocytes and small Lymphocytes. Large granular Lymphocytes include natural killer cells (NK cells).
Leukocytes	White blood cells are cells of the immune system defending the body against both infectious disease and foreign materials. Five different and diverse types of Leukocytes exist, but they are all produced and derived from a multipotent cell in the bone marrow known as a hematopoietic stem cell. Leukocytes are found throughout the body, including the blood and lymphatic system.
Angiogenesis	Angiogenesis is the physiological process involving the growth of new blood vessels from pre-existing vessels. Though there has been some debate over terminology, vasculogenesis is the term used for spontaneous blood-vessel formation, and intussusception is the term for new blood vessel formation by splitting off existing ones.

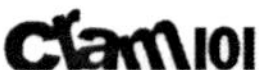

Angiogenesis is a normal and vital process in growth and development, as well as in wound healing and in granulation tissue.

Fibrosis

Fibrosis is the formation or development of excess fibrous connective tissue in an organ or tissue as a reparative or reactive process, as opposed to a formation of fibrous tissue as a normal constituent of an organ or tissue. Scarring is confluent Fibrosis that obliterates the architecture of the underlying organ or tissue.

The term is also sometimes used to describe a normal healing process, but this usage is less common.

· Pulmonary Fibrosis

· Idiopathic pulmonary Fibrosis

· Cirrhosis (liver)

· Endomyocardial Fibrosis

· Mediastinal Fibrosis

· MyeloFibrosis

· Retroperitoneal Fibrosis

· Progressive massive Fibrosis; a complication of coal workers` pneumoconiosis

· Nephrogenic systemic Fibrosis

· Crohn`s Disease (intestine)

· Keloid (skin)

· Old myocardial infarction (heart)

· Scleroderma/systemic sclerosis (skin, lungs)

·

Protein

Proteins are organic compounds made of amino acids arranged in a linear chain and folded into a globular form. The amino acids in a polymer chain are joined together by the peptide bonds between the carboxyl and amino groups of adjacent amino acid residues. The sequence of amino acids in a protein is defined by the sequence of a gene, which is encoded in the genetic code.

Cystic fibrosis

Cystic fibrosis (also known as Cystic fibrosis, mucovoidosis,) is a genetic disorder known to be an inherited disease of the secretory glands, including the glands that make mucus and sweat. The hallmarks of Cystic fibrosis are salty tasting skin, normal appetite but poor growth and poor weight gain, excess mucus production, frequent chest infections and coughing/shortness of breath. Males can be infertile due to the condition Congenital absence of the vas deferens.

Monitoring

To monitor or Monitoring generally means to be aware of the state of a system. Below are specific examples:

· to observe a situation for any changes which may occur over time, using a monitor or measuring device of some sort:

· Baby monitor, medical monitor, Heart rate monitor

· BioMonitoring

· Cure Monitoring for composite materials manufacturing

· Deformation Monitoring

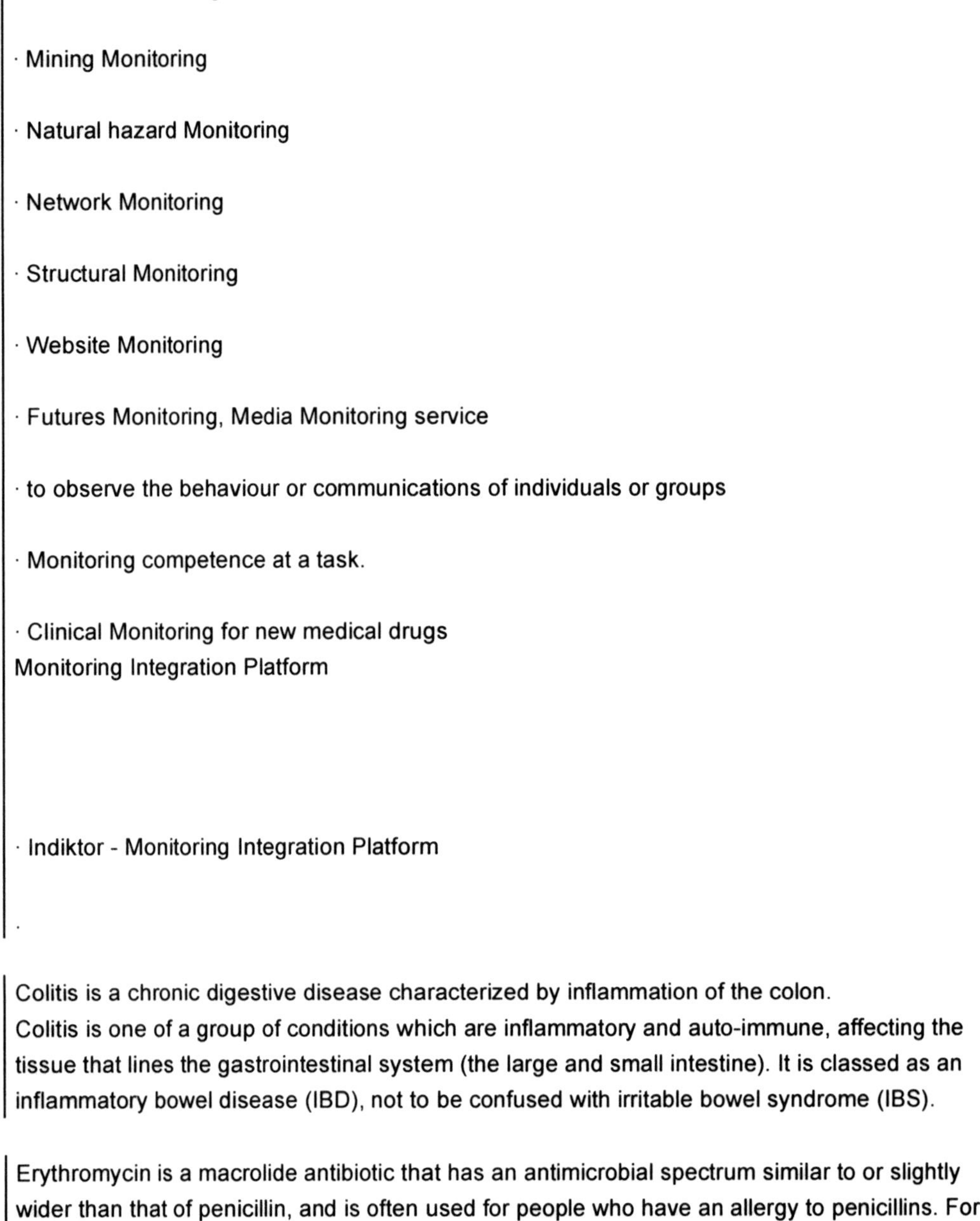

· Election Monitoring

· Mining Monitoring

· Natural hazard Monitoring

· Network Monitoring

· Structural Monitoring

· Website Monitoring

· Futures Monitoring, Media Monitoring service

· to observe the behaviour or communications of individuals or groups

· Monitoring competence at a task.

· Clinical Monitoring for new medical drugs
Monitoring Integration Platform

· Indiktor - Monitoring Integration Platform

·

Colitis

Colitis is a chronic digestive disease characterized by inflammation of the colon. Colitis is one of a group of conditions which are inflammatory and auto-immune, affecting the tissue that lines the gastrointestinal system (the large and small intestine). It is classed as an inflammatory bowel disease (IBD), not to be confused with irritable bowel syndrome (IBS).

Erythromycin

Erythromycin is a macrolide antibiotic that has an antimicrobial spectrum similar to or slightly wider than that of penicillin, and is often used for people who have an allergy to penicillins. For respiratory tract infections, it has better coverage of atypical organisms, including mycoplasma and Legionellosis. It was first marketed by Eli Lilly and Company, and it is today commonly known as EES (Erythromycin ethylsuccinate, an ester prodrug that is commonly administered).

Ulcerative colitis	Ulcerative colitis (Colitis ulcerosa, Ulcerative colitis) is a form of inflammatory bowel disease (IBD). Ulcerative colitis is a form of colitis, a disease of the intestine, specifically the large intestine or colon, that includes characteristic ulcers, or open sores, in the colon. The main symptom of active disease is usually constant diarrhea mixed with blood, of gradual onset.
Usual interstitial pneumonia	Usual interstitial pneumonia, commonly abbreviated Usual interstitial pneumonia, is the name of a histopathological pattern seen in diffuse lung diseases, i.e. interstitial lung diseases. It is classified as an idiopathic interstitial pneumonia, and may be idiopathic, i.e. the cause is unknown, or due to a known cause, e.g. asbestos exposure. The hallmarks of Usual interstitial pneumonia are interstitial inflammation, i.e. inflammation of the alveolar walls, and fibrosis (scarring).
Bronchodilator	A Bronchodilator is a substance that dilates the bronchi and bronchioles, decreasing airway resistance and thereby facilitating airflow. Bronchodilators may be endogenous (originating naturally within the body), or they may be medications administered for the treatment of breathing difficulties. They are most useful in obstructive lung diseases, of which asthma and chronic obstructive pulmonary disease are the most common conditions.
Hyperalgesia	Hyperalgesia is an increased sensitivity to pain, which may be caused by damage to nociceptors or peripheral nerves. Temporary increased sensitivity to pain also occurs as part of sickness behavior, the evolved response to infection. Hyperalgesia can be experienced in focal, discrete areas, or as a more diffuse, body-wide form.
Anti-inflammatory	Anti-inflammatory refers to the property of a substance or treatment that reduces inflammation. Anti-inflammatory drugs make up about half of analgesics, remedying pain by reducing inflammation as opposed to opioids which affect the brain. Steroids Many steroids, specifically glucocorticoids, reduce inflammation or swelling by binding to cortisol receptors.
Glucocorticoid	Glucocorticoids are a class of steroid hormones that bind to the Glucocorticoid receptor (GR), which is present in almost every vertebrate animal cell. The name Glucocorticoid derives from their role in the regulation of the metabolism of glucose, their synthesis in the adrenal cortex, and their steroidal structure .

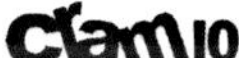

	GCs are part of the feedback mechanism in the immune system that turns immune activity (inflammation) down.
Chronic obstructive pulmonary disease	Chronic obstructive pulmonary disease refers to chronic bronchitis and emphysema, a pair of two commonly co-existing diseases of the lungs in which the airways become narrowed. This leads to a limitation of the flow of air to and from the lungs causing shortness of breath. In contrast to asthma, the limitation of airflow is poorly reversible and usually gets progressively worse over time.
Obstructive lung disease	Obstructive lung disease is a category of respiratory disease characterized by airway obstruction. MeSH includes the following in this category: · Asthma · Bronchitis · Chronic obstructive pulmonary disease Cystic fibrosis is sometimes also included in this category. FEV1/FVC ratio is usually decreased.
Duffy antigen	The Duffy antigen is a protein located on the surface of red blood cells and is named after the patient in which it was discovered. In humans, this protein is encoded by the Duffy antigenRC gene. The protein encoded by this gene is a glycosylated membrane protein and a non-specific receptor for several chemokines.
Dyspnea	Dyspnea , also called shortness of breath (SOB) or air hunger, is a debilitating symptom that is the experience of unpleasant or uncomfortable respiratory sensations. It is a common symptom of numerous medical disorders, particularly those involving the cardiovascular and respiratory systems; Dyspnea on exertion is the most common presenting complaint for people with respiratory impairment.

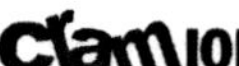

Dyspnea has been more specifically defined by the American Thoracic Society as the `subjective experience of breathing discomfort that consists of qualitatively distinct sensations that vary in intensity.

Emphysema

Emphysema is a lung disease, characterized by an abnormal, permanent enlargement of air spaces distal to the terminal bronchioles. The disease is coupled with the destruction of walls, but without obvious fibrosis. It is often caused by exposure to toxic chemicals, including long-term exposure to tobacco smoke.

Hypoxia

Hypoxia, is a pathological condition in which the body as a whole (generalized hypoxia) or a region of the body (tissue hypoxia) is deprived of adequate oxygen supply. Variations in arterial oxygen concentrations can be part of the normal physiology, for example, during strenuous physical exercise. A mismatch between oxygen supply and its demand at the cellular level may result in a hypoxic condition.

Artery

The arterial system is the higher-pressure portion of the circulatory system. Arterial pressure varies between the peak pressure during heart contraction, called the systolic pressure, and the minimum, or diastolic pressure between contractions, when the heart expands and refills. This pressure variation within the Artery produces the pulse which is observable in any Artery, and reflects heart activity.

Coronary artery disease

(Coronary artery disease or atherosclerotic heart disease) is the end result of the accumulation of atheromatous plaques within the walls of the coronary arteries that supply the myocardium (the muscle of the heart) with oxygen and nutrients. It is sometimes also called coronary heart disease (CHD), although Coronary artery disease is the most common cause of CHD, it is not the only one.

Coronary artery disease is the leading cause of death worldwide.

Corticosteroid

Corticosteroids are a class of steroid hormones that are produced in the adrenal cortex. Corticosteroids are involved in a wide range of physiologic systems such as stress response, immune response and regulation of inflammation, carbohydrate metabolism, protein catabolism, blood electrolyte levels, and behavior.

· Glucocorticoids such as cortisol control carbohydrate, fat and protein metabolism and are anti-inflammatory by preventing phospholipid release, decreasing eosinophil action and a number of other mechanisms.

· Mineralocorticoids such as aldosterone control electrolyte and water levels, mainly by promoting sodium retention in the kidney.

Some common natural hormones are corticosterone ($C_{21}H_{30}O_4$), cortisone ($C_{21}H_{28}O_5$, 17-hydroxy-11-dehydrocorticosterone) and aldosterone.

Connective tissue

Connective tissue is a form of fibrous tissue. It is one of the four types of tissue in traditional classifications (the others being epithelial, muscle, and nervous tissue).

Collagen is the main protein of Connective tissue in animals and the most abundant protein in mammals, making up about 25% of the total protein content.

Fiber types as follows:

· collagenous fibers

· elastic fibers

· Bone Marrow

Various Connective tissue conditions have been identified; these can be both inherited and environmental.

· Marfan syndrome - a genetic disease causing abnormal fibrillin.

· Scurvy - caused by a dietary deficiency in vitamin C, leading to abnormal collagen.

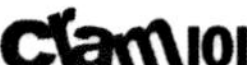

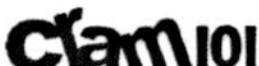

· Ehlers-Danlos syndrome - deficient type III collagen- a genetic disease causing progressive deterioration of collagens, with different EDS types affecting different sites in the body, such as joints, heart valves, organ walls, arterial walls, etc.

· Loeys-Dietz syndrome - a genetic disease related to Marfan syndrome, with an emphasis on vascular deterioration.

· Pseudoxanthoma elasticum - an autosomal recessive hereditary disease, caused by calcification and fragmentation of elastic fibres, affecting the skin, the eyes and the cardiovascular system.

· Systemic lupus erythematosus - a chronic, multisystem, inflammatory disorder of probable autoimmune etiology, occurring predominantly in young women.

· Osteogenesis imperfecta (brittle bone disease) - caused by insufficient production of good quality collagen to produce healthy, strong bones.

· Fibrodysplasia ossificans progressiva - disease of the Connective tissue, caused by a defective gene which turns Connective tissue into bone.

· Spontaneous pneumothorax - collapsed lung, believed to be related to subtle abnormalities in Connective tissue.

· Sarcoma - a neoplastic process originating within Connective tissue.

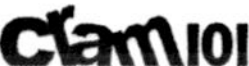

Chapter 6. Triggers of Asthma and COPD

Atherosclerosis	Atherosclerosis is a condition in which an artery wall thickens as the result of a build-up of fatty materials such as cholesterol. It is a syndrome affecting arterial blood vessels, a chronic inflammatory response in the walls of arteries, in large part due to the accumulation of macrophage white blood cells and promoted by low-density lipoproteins (plasma proteins that carry cholesterol and triglycerides) without adequate removal of fats and cholesterol from the macrophages by functional high density lipoproteins (HDL), . It is commonly referred to as a hardening or furring of the arteries.
Cladosporium	Cladosporium is a genus of fungi including some of the most common indoor and outdoor molds. It produces olive-green to brown or black colonies, and its dark-pigmented conidia are formed in simple or branching chains. The many species of Cladosporium are commonly found on living and dead plant material.
Allergen	An Allergen is a nonparasitic antigen capable of stimulating a type-I hypersensitivity reaction in atopic individuals. Most humans mount significant Immunoglobulin E responses only as a defense against parasitic infections. However, some individuals mount an IgE response against common environmental antigens.
Asthma	Asthma is characterized by a predisposition to chronic inflammation of the lungs in which the airways (bronchi) are reversibly narrowed. Asthma affects 7% of the population of the United States, 6.5% of British people and a total of 300 million worldwide. During Asthma attacks (exacerbations of Asthma), the smooth muscle cells in the bronchi constrict, the airways become inflamed and swollen, and breathing becomes difficult.
Calcium channel	A Calcium channel is an ion channel which displays selective permeabiltiy to calcium ions. It is sometimes synonymous as voltage-dependent calcium channel, although there are also ligand-gated calcium channels. Comparison tables The following tables explain gating, gene, location and function of different types of calcium channels, both voltage and ligand-gated.

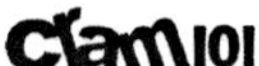

Catarrh	Catarrh is a disorder of inflammation of the mucous membranes. It can result in a thick exudate of mucus and white blood cells caused by the swelling of the mucous membranes in the head in response to an infection. It is a symptom usually associated with the common cold and chesty coughs, but can also be found in patients with infections of the adenoids, middle ear, sinus or tonsils.
Disease	A disease or medical condition is an abnormal condition of an organism that impairs bodily functions, associated with specific symptoms and signs. It may be caused by external factors, such as invading organisms, or it may be caused by internal dysfunctions, such as autoimmune diseases. In human beings, \`disease\` is often used more broadly to refer to any condition that causes pain, dysfunction, distress, social problems, and/or death to the person afflicted, or similar problems for those in contact with the person.
Fever	Fever is a frequent medical sign that describes an increase in internal body temperature to levels above normal. Fever is most accurately characterized as a temporary elevation in the body's thermoregulatory set-point, usually by about 1-2 °C (1.8-3.6 °F). Fever is caused by an elevation in the thermoregulatory set-point, causing typical body temperature (generally and problematically considered to be 37 °C or 98.6 °F) to rise, and effector mechanisms are enacted as a result.
Protein	Proteins are organic compounds made of amino acids arranged in a linear chain and folded into a globular form. The amino acids in a polymer chain are joined together by the peptide bonds between the carboxyl and amino groups of adjacent amino acid residues. The sequence of amino acids in a protein is defined by the sequence of a gene, which is encoded in the genetic code.
Constipation	Constipation, costiveness,) experiences hard feces (faeces) that are difficult to expel. This usually happens because the colon absorbs too much water from the food. If the food moves through the gastro-intestinal tract too slowly, the colon may absorb too much water, resulting in feces that are dry and hard.
Atopy	Atopy or atopic syndrome is an allergic hypersensitivity affecting parts of the body not in direct contact with the allergen. It may involve eczema , allergic conjunctivitis, allergic rhinitis and asthma. There appears to be a strong hereditary component.
Factor XII	Hageman factor is a plasma protein , an enzyme (EC 3.4.21.38) of the serine protease (or serine endopeptidase) class. In humans, Factor XII is encoded by the F12 gene.

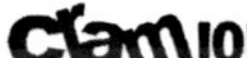

	It is part of the coagulation cascade and activates factor XI and prekallikrein.
Functional residual capacity	Functional residual capacity is the volume of air present in the lungs at the end of passive expiration. At Functional residual capacity, the elastic recoil forces of the lungs and chest wall are equal but opposite and there is no exertion by the diaphragm or other respiratory muscles. FRC is the sum of Expiratory Reserve Volume (ERV) and Residual Volume (RV) and measures approximately 2400 ml in a 70 kg, average-sized male.
Growth factor	A Growth factor is a naturally occurring substance capable of stimulating cellular growth, proliferation and cellular differentiation. Usually it is a protein or a steroid hormone. Growth factors are important for regulating a variety of cellular processes.
Leukocytes	White blood cells are cells of the immune system defending the body against both infectious disease and foreign materials. Five different and diverse types of Leukocytes exist, but they are all produced and derived from a multipotent cell in the bone marrow known as a hematopoietic stem cell. Leukocytes are found throughout the body, including the blood and lymphatic system.
Neuroendocrine	Neuroendocrine [IPA nÊŠÉ™roÊŠËˆÉ›ndÉ™krÉªn] cells are cells that release a hormone into the circulating blood in response to a neural stimulus. These hormones may be amines, neuropeptides, or specialized amino acids. They package the hormones in vesicles and send these packages via long processes to blood vessels.
Pollen	Pollen is a fine to coarse powder containing the microgametophytes of seed plants, which produce the male gametes (sperm cells). Pollen grains have a hard coat that protects the sperm cells during the process of their movement between the stamens to the pistil of flowering plants or from the male cone to the female cone of coniferous plants. When pollen lands on a compatible pistil of flowering plants, it germinates and produces a pollen tube that transfers the sperm to the ovule of a receptive ovary.
Dose	A dose is a quantity of something (chemical, physical, or biological) that may impact an organism biologically; the greater the quantity, the larger the dose. In nutrition, the term is usually applied to how much of a specific nutrient is in a person's diet or in a particular food, meal, or dietary supplement. In medicine, the term is usually applied to the quantity of a drug or other agent administered for therapeutic purposes.
Duffy antigen	The Duffy antigen is a protein located on the surface of red blood cells and is named after the patient in which it was discovered. In humans, this protein is encoded by the Duffy antigenRC gene.

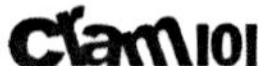

	The protein encoded by this gene is a glycosylated membrane protein and a non-specific receptor for several chemokines.
Inhaler	An Inhaler or puffer is a medical device used for delivering medication into the body via the lungs. It is mainly used in the treatment of asthma and Chronic Obstructive Pulmonary Disease (COPD). To reduce deposition in the mouth and throat, and to reduce the need for precise synchronization of the start of inhalation with actuation of the device, MDIs are sometimes used with a complementary spacer or holding chamber device.
Metered Dose Inhaler	A metered-dose inhaler is a device that delivers a specific amount of medication to the lungs, in the form of a short burst of aerosolized medicine that is inhaled by the patient. It is the most commonly used delivery system for treating asthma, chronic obstructive pulmonary disease (COPD) and other respiratory diseases. The medication in a Metered dose inhaler is most commonly a bronchodilator, corticosteroid or a combination of both for the treatment of asthma and COPD. Other medications less commonly used but also administered by Metered dose inhaler are mast cell stabilizers, such as (cromoglicate or nedocromil).
SNARE	SNARE proteins REceptors` are a large protein superfamily consisting of more than 60 members in yeast and mammalian cells. The primary role of SNARE proteins is to mediate vesicle fusion, that is, the exocytosis of cellular transport vesicles with the cell membrane at the porosome or with a target compartment (such as a lysosome). SNAREs can be divided into two categories: vesicle or v-SNAREs , which are incorporated into the membranes of transport vesicles during budding, and target or t-SNAREs, which are located in the membranes of target compartments.
Artery	The arterial system is the higher-pressure portion of the circulatory system. Arterial pressure varies between the peak pressure during heart contraction, called the systolic pressure, and the minimum, or diastolic pressure between contractions, when the heart expands and refills. This pressure variation within the Artery produces the pulse which is observable in any Artery, and reflects heart activity.
Chronic obstructive pulmonary disease	Chronic obstructive pulmonary disease refers to chronic bronchitis and emphysema, a pair of two commonly co-existing diseases of the lungs in which the airways become narrowed. This leads to a limitation of the flow of air to and from the lungs causing shortness of breath. In contrast to asthma, the limitation of airflow is poorly reversible and usually gets progressively worse over time.

Coronary artery disease	(Coronary artery disease or atherosclerotic heart disease) is the end result of the accumulation of atheromatous plaques within the walls of the coronary arteries that supply the myocardium (the muscle of the heart) with oxygen and nutrients. It is sometimes also called coronary heart disease (CHD), although Coronary artery disease is the most common cause of CHD, it is not the only one. Coronary artery disease is the leading cause of death worldwide.
Corticosteroid	Corticosteroids are a class of steroid hormones that are produced in the adrenal cortex. Corticosteroids are involved in a wide range of physiologic systems such as stress response, immune response and regulation of inflammation, carbohydrate metabolism, protein catabolism, blood electrolyte levels, and behavior. · Glucocorticoids such as cortisol control carbohydrate, fat and protein metabolism and are anti-inflammatory by preventing phospholipid release, decreasing eosinophil action and a number of other mechanisms. · Mineralocorticoids such as aldosterone control electrolyte and water levels, mainly by promoting sodium retention in the kidney. Some common natural hormones are corticosterone ($C_{21}H_{30}O_4$), cortisone ($C_{21}H_{28}O_5$, 17-hydroxy-11-dehydrocorticosterone) and aldosterone.
Defensins	Defensins are small cysteine-rich cationic proteins found in both vertebrates and invertebrates. They are active against bacteria, fungi and many enveloped and nonenveloped viruses. They consist of 18-45 amino acids including six (in vertebrates) to 8 conserved cysteine residues.
Dendritic cell	Dendritic cells are immune cells that form part of the mammalian immune system. Their main function is to process antigen material and present it on the surface to other cells of the immune system, thus functioning as antigen-presenting cells. They act as messengers between the innate and adaptive immunity.

	Dendritic cells are present in small quantities in tissues that are in contact with the external environment, mainly the skin (where there is a specialized Dendritic cell type called Langerhans cells) and the inner lining of the nose, lungs, stomach and intestines. They can also be found in an immature state in the blood.
Ejection fraction	In cardiovascular physiology, ejection fraction is the fraction of blood pumped out of the right and left ventricles with each heart beat. The term ejection fraction applies to both the right and left ventricles; one can speak equally of the left ventricular ejection fraction and the right ventricular ejection fraction. RVEF and LVEF may vary widely from one another incumbent upon physiologic state.
Pathophysiology	Pathophysiology is the study of the changes of normal mechanical, physical, and biochemical functions, either caused by a disease, it is the branch of medicine which deals with any disturbances of body functions, caused by disease or prodromal symptoms. An alternate definition is `the study of the biological and physical manifestations of disease as they correlate with the underlying abnormalities and physiological disturbances.` The study of pathology and the study of Pathophysiology often involves substantial overlap in diseases and processes, but pathology emphasizes direct observations, while Pathophysiology emphasizes quantifiable measurements.
Salbutamol	Salbutamol (INN) or albuterol (USAN) is a short-acting β_2-adrenergic receptor agonist used for the relief of bronchospasm in conditions such as asthma and chronic obstructive pulmonary disease. It is marketed by GlaxoSmithKline as Ventolin, Aerolin or Ventorlin depending on the market; by Cipla as Asthalin; by Schering-Plough as Proventil and by Teva as ProAir. Generic names are currently not available in the U.S. because of a federal ban on the use of CFCs.
Salmeterol	Salmeterol is a long-acting beta2-adrenergic receptor agonist drug that is currently prescribed for the treatment of asthma and chronic obstructive pulmonary disease (COPD). It is currently available as a metered-dose inhaler (MDI) or a proprietary `disk-styled` inhaler that releases a powdered form of the drug. It is a long acting beta-adrenoceptor agonist (LABA), usually only prescribed for severe persistent asthma following previous treatment with a short-acting beta agonist such as salbutamol and is prescribed concurrently with a corticosteroid, such as beclomethasone.
Terbutaline	Terbutaline (trade names Brethine, Bricanyl, or Brethaire) is a β_2-adrenergic receptor agonist, used as a fast-acting bronchodilator (often used as a short-term asthma treatment) and as a tocolytic to delay premature labour. The inhaled form of Terbutaline starts working within 15 minutes and can last up to 6 hours.

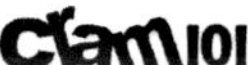

	Terbutaline as a treatment for premature labour is an off-label use not approved by the FDA. It is a pregnancy category `B` medication and is routinely prescribed to stop contractions.
Subclinical infection	A Subclinical infection is the asymptomatic (without apparent sign) carrying of an (infection) by an individual of an agent (microbe, intestinal parasite,) that usually is a pathogen causing illness, at least in some individuals. Many pathogens spread by being silently carried in this way by some of their host population. Such infections occur both in humans and nonhuman animals.
Volume	The Volume of any solid, liquid, gas, plasma, or vacuum is how much three-dimensional space it occupies, often quantified numerically. One-dimensional figures (such as lines) and two-dimensional shapes (such as squares) are assigned zero Volume in the three-dimensional space. Volume is commonly presented in units such as cubic meters, cubic centimeters, liters, or milliliters.
Platelet	Platelets, or thrombocytes , are small, irregularly-shaped anuclear cells , 2-3 Âµm in diameter, which are derived from fragmentation of precursor megakaryocytes. The average lifespan of a Platelet is between 8 and 12 days. Platelets play a fundamental role in hemostasis and are a natural source of growth factors.
Allergic bronchopulmonary aspergillosis	In medicine, Allergic bronchopulmonary aspergillosis (ABPA) is a condition characterised by an exaggerated response of the immune system (a hypersensitivity response) to the fungus Aspergillus (most commonly Aspergillus fumigatus). It occurs most often in patients with asthma or cystic fibrosis. Aspergillus spores are ubiquitous in soil and are commonly found in the sputum of healthy individuals.
Diagnosis	In medicine, diagnosis (plural, diagnoses) is the process of identifying a medical condition or disease by its signs, symptoms, and from the results of various diagnostic procedures. The conclusion reached through this process is called a diagnosis. The term `diagnostic criteria` designates the combination of signs, symptoms, and test results that allows the health care practitioner to ascertain the diagnosis of the respective disease.
Presentation	Presentation is the practice of showing and explaining the content of a topic to an audience or learner. A Presentation program, such as Microsoft PowerPoint, is often used to generate the Presentation content. · BCG diagram: This diagram is extremely useful in marketing, although most people only learn the basics of the diagram at undergraduate level.

Bronchiectasis

Bronchiectasis is a disease that causes localized, irreversible dilation of part of the bronchial tree. It is classified as an obstructive lung disease, along with bronchitis and cystic fibrosis. Involved bronchi are dilated, inflamed, and easily collapsible, resulting in airflow obstruction and impaired clearance of secretions.

Cystic fibrosis

Cystic fibrosis (also known as Cystic fibrosis, mucovoidosis,) is a genetic disorder known to be an inherited disease of the secretory glands, including the glands that make mucus and sweat. The hallmarks of Cystic fibrosis are salty tasting skin, normal appetite but poor growth and poor weight gain, excess mucus production, frequent chest infections and coughing/shortness of breath. Males can be infertile due to the condition Congenital absence of the vas deferens.

Eosinophilia

Eosinophilia is the state of having a high concentration of eosinophils (eosinophil granulocytes) in the blood. The normal concentration is between 0 and 0.5×10^9 eosinophils per litre of blood. Eosinophilia can be reactive (in response to other stimuli such as allergy or infection) or non reactive.

Occupational asthma

Occupational asthma is an occupational condition defined as:

`a disease characterized by variable airflow limitation and/or airway hyper-responsiveness due to causes and conditions attributable to a particular occupational environment and not stimuli encountered outside the workplace`.

Asthma is defined as a respiratory disease caused by narrowing of the air passages. It is synonymous with difficulty in breathing, tightness of chest, nasal irritation, coughing and wheezing.

Biocide

A Biocide is a chemical substance capable of killing living organisms, usually in a selective way. Biocides are commonly used in medicine, agriculture, forestry, and in industry where they prevent the fouling of water and oil pipelines. Some substances used as Biocides are also employed as anti-fouling agents or disinfectants under other circumstances: chlorine, for example, is used as a short-life Biocide in industrial water treatment but as a disinfectant in swimming pools.

Pathology

Pathology is the study and diagnosis of disease through examination of organs, tissues, bodily fluids, and whole bodies (autopsies). The term also encompasses the related scientific study of disease processes, called General Pathology.

Medical Pathology is divided in two main branches, Anatomical Pathology and Clinical Pathology.

Womanhood

Womanhood is the period in a female`s life after she has transitioned from girlhood, at least physically, having passed the age of menarche. Many cultures have rites of passage to symbolize a woman`s coming of age, such as confirmation in some branches of Christianity, bat mitzvah in Judaism, or even just the custom of a special celebration for a certain birthday (generally between 12 and 21).

The word woman can be used generally, to mean any female human, or specifically, to mean an adult female human as contrasted with girl.

Lung

The Lung or pulmonary system is the essential respiration organ in all air-breathing animals, including most tetrapods, a few fish and a few snails. In mammals and the more complex life forms, the two Lungs are located in the chest on either side of the heart. Their principal function is to transport oxygen from the atmosphere into the bloodstream, and to release carbon dioxide from the bloodstream into the atmosphere.

Obstructive lung disease

Obstructive lung disease is a category of respiratory disease characterized by airway obstruction.

MeSH includes the following in this category:

· Asthma

· Bronchitis

· Chronic obstructive pulmonary disease

Cystic fibrosis is sometimes also included in this category.

FEV1/FVC ratio is usually decreased.

Respiratory tract infection

Respiratory tract infection refers to any of a number of infectious diseases involving the respiratory tract. An infection of this type is normally further classified as an upper respiratory tract infection or a lower respiratory tract infection. Lower respiratory infections, such as pneumonia, tend to be far more serious conditions than upper respiratory infections, such as the common cold.

Chapter 6. Triggers of Asthma and COPD

Viral	The term Viral is used to describe anything related to viruses. Viral may also mean: · .
Rhinovirus	Human Rhinovirus A Human Rhinovirus B Human Rhinovirus C Rhinovirus was a genus of the Picornaviridae family of viruses. It has been now merged into Enteroviruses, a group of Picornaviridae that includes Poliovirus, Coxsackie A virus, and Hepatitis A. Rhinoviruses are the most common viral infective agents in humans, and a causative agent of the common cold. It is lytic in nature.
Allergic rhinitis	Allergic rhinitis, pollenosis or hay fever is an allergic inflammation of the nasal airways. It occurs when an allergen such as pollen or dust is inhaled by an individual with a sensitized immune system, and triggers antibody production. The specific antibody is immunoglobulin E (IgE) which binds to mast cells and basophils containing histamine.
Bronchiolitis	Bronchiolitis is inflammation of the bronchioles, the smallest air passages of the lungs. This inflammation is usually caused by viruses. The term usually refers to acute viral Bronchiolitis, a common disease in infancy.
Lymphocyte	A Lymphocyte is a type of white blood cell in the vertebrate immune system. Under the microscope, Lymphocytes can be divided into large granular Lymphocytes and small Lymphocytes. Large granular Lymphocytes include natural killer cells (NK cells).

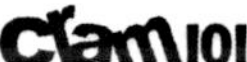

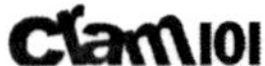

Paracetamol	Paracetamol or acetaminophen) is a widely used over-the-counter analgesic (pain reliever) and antipyretic (fever reducer). However, its effectiveness alone as an antipyretic has been questioned. It is commonly used for the relief of headaches, and other minor aches and pains, and is a major ingredient in numerous cold and flu remedies.
Syndrome	In medicine and psychology, the term syndrome refers to the association of several clinically recognizable features, signs (observed by a physician), symptoms (reported by the patient), phenomena or characteristics that often occur together, so that the presence of one feature alerts the physician to the presence of the others. In recent decades the term has been used outside of medicine to refer to a combination of phenomena seen in association. The term syndrome derives from its Greek roots and means literally `run together`, as the features do.
Immunity	Immunity is a biological term that describes a state of having sufficient biological defenses to avoid infection, disease, or other unwanted biological invasion. Immunity involves both specific and non-specific components. The non-specific components act either as barriers or as eliminators of wide range of pathogens irrespective of antigenic specificity.
Inflammation	Inflammation is the complex biological response of vascular tissues to harmful stimuli, such as pathogens, damaged cells, or irritants. Inflammation is a protective attempt by the organism to remove the injurious stimuli as well as initiate the healing process for the tissue. Inflammation is not a synonym for infection.
Primary	In medicine, the reporting of symptoms by a patient may have significant psychological motivators. Psychologists sometimes categorize these motivators into primary or secondary gain. primary gain is internally good; motivationally.
Macrophages	Macrophages are white blood cells within tissues, produced by the division of monocytes. Human Macrophages are about 21 micrometres (0.00083 in) in diameter. Monocytes and Macrophages are phagocytes, acting in both non-specific defense (innate immunity) as well as to help initiate specific defense mechanisms (adaptive immunity) of vertebrate animals.
Natural killer cells	Natural killer cells are a type of cytotoxic lymphocyte that constitute a major component of the innate immune system. NK cells play a major role in the rejection of tumors and cells infected by viruses. They kill cells by releasing small cytoplasmic granules of proteins called perforin and granzyme that cause the target cell to die by apoptosis.

Erythromycin	Erythromycin is a macrolide antibiotic that has an antimicrobial spectrum similar to or slightly wider than that of penicillin, and is often used for people who have an allergy to penicillins. For respiratory tract infections, it has better coverage of atypical organisms, including mycoplasma and Legionellosis. It was first marketed by Eli Lilly and Company, and it is today commonly known as EES (Erythromycin ethylsuccinate, an ester prodrug that is commonly administered).
Interferon	Interferons (IFNs) are proteins made and released by lymphocytes in response to the presence of pathogens--such as viruses, bacteria, or parasites--or tumor cells. They allow communication between cells to trigger the protective defenses of the immune system that eradicate pathogens or tumors. Interferons belong to the large class of glycoproteins known as cytokines.
Mometasone furoate	Mometasone furoate (also referred to as mometasone) is a glucocorticoid steroid. It is used in the treatment of inflammatory skin disorders (such as eczema and psoriasis), allergic rhinitis (such as hay fever), and asthma for patients unresponsive to less potent corticosteroids. In terms of steroid strength, it is more potent than hydrocortisone, and less potent than dexamethasone.
Type I interferons	Human type I interferons comprise a vast and growing group of IFN proteins. All type I IFNs bind to a specific cell surface receptor complex known as the IFN-α receptor (IFNAR) that consists of IFNAR1 and IFNAR2 chains. Homologous molecules to type I IFNs are found in many species, including all mammals, and some have been identified in birds, reptiles, amphibians and fish species.
Bone	Bones are rigid organs that form part of the endoskeleton of vertebrates. They function to move, support, and protect the various organs of the body, produce red and white blood cells and store minerals. bone tissue is a type of dense connective tissue.

Chapter 6. Triggers of Asthma and COPD

Keratinocyte	Keratinocytes are the predominant cell type in the epidermis, the outermost layer of the human skin, constituting 95% of the cells found there. Those keratinocytes found in the basal layer (Stratum germinativum) of the skin are sometimes referred to as "basal cells" or "basal keratinocytes". The primary function of keratinocytes is the formation of a barrier against environmental damage such as pathogens (bacteria, fungi, parasites, viruses) heat, UV radiation and water loss.
Metabolism	Metabolism is the set of chemical reactions that happen in living organisms to maintain life. These processes allow organisms to grow and reproduce, maintain their structures, and respond to their environments. Metabolism is usually divided into two categories.
Monocyte	Monocyte is a type of white blood cell, part of the human body`s immune system. Monocytes have two main functions in the immune system: (1) replenish resident macrophages and dendritic cells under normal states, and (2) in response to inflammation signals, Monocytes can move quickly (approx. 8-12 hours) to sites of infection in the tissues and divide/differentiate into macrophages and dendritic cells to elicit an immune response.
Mast cell	A Mast cell is a resident cell of several types of tissues and contains many granules rich in histamine and heparin. Although best known for their role in allergy and anaphylaxis, Mast cells play an important protective role as well, being intimately involved in wound healing and defense against pathogens. Mast cells were first described by Paul Ehrlich in his 1878 doctoral thesis on the basis of their unique staining characteristics and large granules.
Mycoplasma pneumonia	Mycoplasma pneumonia is a form of bacterial pneumonia which is caused by the bacteria species Mycoplasma pneumoniae. Disease from mycoplasma is usually mild to moderate in severity. The symptoms are usually mild enough that the patient may remain ambulatory throughout the illness.
Gas exchange	Gas exchange takes place at a respiratory surface--a boundary between the external environment and the interior of the organism. For unicellular organisms the respiratory surface is governed by Fick`s law, which determines that respiratory surfaces must have: · a large surface area · a thin permeable surface

· a moist exchange surface.

Many also have a mechanism to maximise the diffusion gradient by replenishing the source and/or sink.

Control of respiration is due to rhythmical breathing generated by the phrenic nerve in order to stimulate contraction and relaxation of the diaphragm during inspiration and expiration.

Colitis

Colitis is a chronic digestive disease characterized by inflammation of the colon.
Colitis is one of a group of conditions which are inflammatory and auto-immune, affecting the tissue that lines the gastrointestinal system (the large and small intestine). It is classed as an inflammatory bowel disease (IBD), not to be confused with irritable bowel syndrome (IBS).

Immunology

Immunology is a broad branch of biomedical science that covers the study of all aspects of the immune system in all organisms. It deals with, among other things, the physiological functioning of the immune system in states of both health and disease; malfunctions of the immune system in immunological disorders (autoimmune diseases, hypersensitivities, immune deficiency, transplant rejection); the physical, chemical and physiological characteristics of the components of the immune system in vitro, in situ, and in vivo. Immunology has applications in several disciplines of science, and as such is further divided.

Ulcerative colitis

Ulcerative colitis (Colitis ulcerosa, Ulcerative colitis) is a form of inflammatory bowel disease (IBD). Ulcerative colitis is a form of colitis, a disease of the intestine, specifically the large intestine or colon, that includes characteristic ulcers, or open sores, in the colon. The main symptom of active disease is usually constant diarrhea mixed with blood, of gradual onset.

Usual interstitial pneumonia

Usual interstitial pneumonia, commonly abbreviated Usual interstitial pneumonia, is the name of a histopathological pattern seen in diffuse lung diseases, i.e. interstitial lung diseases. It is classified as an idiopathic interstitial pneumonia, and may be idiopathic, i.e. the cause is unknown, or due to a known cause, e.g. asbestos exposure.
The hallmarks of Usual interstitial pneumonia are interstitial inflammation, i.e. inflammation of the alveolar walls, and fibrosis (scarring).

Omalizumab

Omalizumab (Xolair, Genentech / Novartis) is a humanized antibody drug approved for patients with moderate-to-severe or severe allergic asthma, which is caused by hypersensitivity reactions to certain harmless environmental substances. Omalizumab`s cost is high ($10,000 to $30,000 per year), as compared to other drugs used for asthma, and hence Omalizumab is mainly prescribed for patients with severe, persistent asthma, which cannot be controlled even with high doses of corticosteroids. Like other protein and antibody drugs, Omalizumab causes anaphylaxis (a life-threatening systemic allergic reaction) in 1 to 2 patients per 1,000.

Epithelial-mesenchymal transition

Epithelial-mesenchymal transition is a hypothesized program of development of biological cells characterized by loss of cell adhesion, repression of E-cadherin expression, and increased cell mobility. Epithelial mesenchymal transition may be essential for numerous developmental processes including mesoderm formation and neural tube formation.

Induction

Several oncogenic pathways (peptide growth factors, Src, Ras, Ets, integrin, Wnt/beta-catenin and Notch) may induce Epithelial mesenchymal transition. In particular, Ras-MAPK has been shown to activate two related transcription factors known as Snail and Slug.

Military psychiatrist

A Military psychiatrist is usually a professional that deals with the treatment of military personnel and officers studying the psychological problems consequent to a real war, a virtual one, Treatment and Strategy Counselling.

Notable Military psychiatrists are or have been:

· Sidney Gottlieb (1918-1999)

· Werner Heyde (1902-1964)

· Friedrich Panse (1899-1973)

· W. H. R. Rivers (1864-1922)

· Ernst Rüdin (1874-1952)

	· Simon Wessely (?-living) `
Medical ventilator	A Medical ventilator may be defined as any machine designed to mechanically move breatheable air into and out of the lungs, to provide the mechanism of breathing for a patient who is physically unable to breathe
Vascular endothelial growth factor	Vascular endothelial growth factor is a signal protein produced by cells that stimulates the growth of new blood vessels. It is part of the system that restores the oxygen supply to tissues when blood circulation is inadequate. Vascular endothelial growth factor's normal function is to create new blood vessels during embryonic development, new blood vessels after injury, muscle following exercise, and new vessels (collateral circulation) to bypass blocked vessels.
Epidemic	In epidemiology, an Epidemic occurs when new cases of a certain disease, in a given human population, and during a given period, substantially exceed what is `expected,` based on recent experience . (An epizootic is the analogous circumstance within an animal population). In recent usages, the disease is not required to be communicable; examples include cancer or heart disease.
Excited delirium	Excited delirium is a controversial term used to explain deaths of individuals in police custody, in which the person being arrested or restrained shows some combination of agitation, violent or bizarre behavior, insensitivity to pain, elevated body temperature
Necrosis	Necrosis is the premature death of cells and living tissue. Necrosis is caused by factors external to the cell or tissue, such as infection, toxins, or trauma. This is in contrast to apoptosis, which is a naturally occurring cause of cellular death.
Bronchodilator	A Bronchodilator is a substance that dilates the bronchi and bronchioles, decreasing airway resistance and thereby facilitating airflow. Bronchodilators may be endogenous (originating naturally within the body), or they may be medications administered for the treatment of breathing difficulties. They are most useful in obstructive lung diseases, of which asthma and chronic obstructive pulmonary disease are the most common conditions.

Intervention	An intervention is an orchestrated attempt by one, or often many, people (usually family and friends) to get someone to seek professional help with an addiction or some kind of traumatic event or crisis, or other serious problem. The term intervention is most often used when the traumatic event involves addiction to drugs or other items. intervention can also refer to the act of using a technique within a therapy session.
Strength training	Strength training is the use of resistance to muscular contraction to build the strength, anaerobic endurance and size of skeletal muscles. There are many different methods of Strength training, the most common being the use of gravity or elastic/hydraulic forces to oppose muscle contraction.
Surgery	Surgery is the branch of medicine that deals with the physical manipulation of a bodily structure to diagnose, prevent, a 16th century French surgeon, stated that there were five reasons to perform Surgery: `To eliminate that which is superfluous, restore that which has been dislocated, separate that which has been united, join that which has been divided and repair the defects of nature.` Since human beings first learned to make and handle tools, they have employed their talents to develop surgical techniques, each time more sophisticated than the last; however, up until the industrial revolution, surgeons were incapable of overcoming the three principal obstacles which had plagued the medical profession from its infancy -- bleeding, pain and infection. Advances in these fields have transformed Surgery from a risky `art` into a scientific discipline capable of treating many diseases and conditions.
Hypertension	Hypertension is a chronic medical condition in which the blood pressure is elevated. It is also referred to as high blood pressure or shortened to HT, HTN or HPN. The word `Hypertension`, by itself, normally refers to systemic, arterial Hypertension. Hypertension can be classified as either essential (primary) or secondary.
Pulmonary hypertension	In medicine, Pulmonary hypertension (Pulmonary hypertension or Pulmonary hypertensionT) is an increase in blood pressure in the pulmonary artery, pulmonary vein, together known as the lung vasculature, leading to shortness of breath, dizziness, fainting, and other symptoms, all of which are exacerbated by exertion. Pulmonary hypertension can be a severe disease with a markedly decreased exercise tolerance and heart failure. It was first identified by Dr. Ernst von Romberg in 1891.
Pollutant	A Pollutant is a waste material that pollutes air, water or soil. Three factors determine the severity of a Pollutant: its chemical nature, the concentration and the persistence. Some Pollutants are biodegradable and therefore will not persist in the environment in the long term.

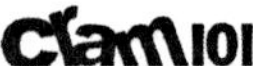

Chapter 6. Triggers of Asthma and COPD

Bronchial hyperresponsiveness	Bronchial hyperresponsiveness (or other combinations with airway or hyperreactivity) is a state characterised by easily triggered bronchospasm (contraction of the bronchioles or small airways). Bronchial hyperresponsiveness can be assessed with a bronchial challenge test. This most often uses products like metacholine or histamine.
Anti-inflammatory	Anti-inflammatory refers to the property of a substance or treatment that reduces inflammation. Anti-inflammatory drugs make up about half of analgesics, remedying pain by reducing inflammation as opposed to opioids which affect the brain. Steroids Many steroids, specifically glucocorticoids, reduce inflammation or swelling by binding to cortisol receptors.
Nonsteroidal anti-inflammatory drugs	Nonsteroidal anti-inflammatory drugs, usually abbreviated to NSAIDs or Nonsteroidal anti inflammatory drugss, are drugs with analgesic and antipyretic (fever-reducing) effects and which have, in higher doses, anti-inflammatory effects (reducing inflammation). The term `nonsteroidal` is used to distinguish these drugs from steroids, which (among a broad range of other effects) have a similar eicosanoid-depressing, anti-inflammatory action. As analgesics, NSAIDs are unusual in that they are non-narcotic.
Desensitization	For telecommunications, desensitization is a form of electromagnetic interference where a radio receiver is unable to receive a weak radio signal that it might otherwise be able to receive when there is no interference. This is caused by a nearby transmitter with a strong signal on a close frequency, which overloads the receiver and makes it unable to fully receive the desired signal. Typical receiver operation is such that the Minimum Detectable Signal (MDS) level is determined by the thermal noise of its electronic components.
Idiopathic	Idiopathic is an adjective used primarily in medicine meaning arising spontaneously or from an obscure or unknown cause. From Greek á¼´διος, idios + πÎ¬θος, pathos (suffering), it means approximately `a disease of its own kind.` It is technically a term from nosology, the classification of disease. For most medical conditions, one or more causes are somewhat understood, but in a certain percentage of people with the condition, the cause may not be readily apparent or characterized.

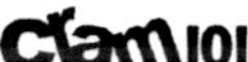

Idiopathic pulmonary fibrosis	Idiopathic pulmonary fibrosis , formerly known as cryptogenic fibrosing alveolitis, is a rare, chronic, progressive interstitial lung disease. Idiopathic pulmonary fibrosis belongs to the subgroup, known as idiopathic interstitial pneumonia (IIP). It is the most common form of the seven distinct IIPs.
Timolol	Timolol maleate is a non-selective beta-adrenergic receptor blocker. In its oral form (Blocadren), it is used to treat high blood pressure and prevent heart attacks, and occasionally to prevent migraine headaches. In its ophthalmic form (brand names Timoptol in Italy; Timoptic), it is used to treat open-angle and occasionally secondary glaucoma by reducing aqueous humour production through blockage of the beta receptors on the ciliary epithelium.
Catecholamines	Catecholamines are sympathomimetic 'fight-or-flight' hormones that are released by the adrenal glands in response to stress. They are part of the sympathetic nervous system. They are called Catecholamines because they contain a catechol group, and are derived from the amino acid tyrosine.
Propranolol	Propranolol is a non-selective beta blocker mainly used in the treatment of hypertension. It was the first successful beta blocker developed. It has been studied for the prophylaxis of migraines in children, but because of limited or inconsistent data, this is not an approved use in the US.
ACE inhibitors	ACE inhibitors or angiotensin-converting enzyme inhibitors, are a group of pharmaceuticals that are used primarily in treatment of hypertension and congestive heart failure, in some cases as the drugs of first choice. ACE inhibitors are used primarily in the treatment of hypertension,though they are also sometimes used in those with cardiac failure, renal disease,or systemic sclerosis This system is activated in response to hypotension, decreased sodium concentration in the distal tubule, decreased blood volume and renal sympathetic nerve stimulation. In such a situation, the kidneys release renin which cleaves the liver-derived angiotensinogen into angiotensin I. Angiotensin I is then converted to angiotensin II via the ACE in the pulmonary circulation as well as in the endothelium of blood vessels in many parts of the body.
Multiple inert gas elimination technique	Multiple inert gas elimination technique is a technique used mainly in pneumology, that involves measuring mixed venous, arterial, and mixed expired concentrations of six infused inert gases, shows a shunt, dead space, and the general ventilation versus blood flow (Va/Q).

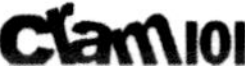

It is a good technique for establishing emphysema or chronic bronchitis.

`.

Anesthetic

An Anesthetic is a drug that causes anesthesia--reversible loss of sensation. These drugs are generally administered to facilitate surgery. A wide variety of drugs are used in modern Anesthetic practice.

Angiotensin

Angiotensin, a protein, causes blood vessels to constrict, and drives blood pressure up. It is part of the renin-Angiotensin system, which is a major target for drugs that lower blood pressure. Angiotensin also stimulates the release of aldosterone from the adrenal cortex.

Captopril

Captopril is an angiotensin-converting enzyme inhibitor used for the treatment of hypertension and some types of congestive heart failure. Captopril was the first ACE inhibitor developed and was considered a breakthrough both because of its novel mechanism of action and also because of the revolutionary development process. Captopril is commonly marketed by Bristol-Myers Squibb under the trade name Capoten.

Local anesthetic

A Local anesthetic is a drug that causes reversible local anesthesia and a loss of nociception. When it is used on specific nerve pathways (nerve block), effects such as analgesia and paralysis can be achieved.

Clinical Local anesthetics belong to one of two classes: aminoamide and aminoester Local anesthetics.

Pilocarpine

Pilocarpine is a parasympathomimetic alkaloid obtained from the leaves of tropical American shrubs from the genus Pilocarpus. It is a non-selective muscarinic receptor agonist in the parasympathetic nervous system, which acts therapeutically at the muscarinic acetylcholine receptor M3 due to its topical application, e.g., in glaucoma and xerostomia.

Uses

Clinical

Pilocarpine has been used in the treatment of chronic open-angle glaucoma and acute angle-closure glaucoma for over 100 years.

Pseudoxanthoma elasticum	Pseudoxanthoma elasticum is a genetic disease that causes fragmentation and mineralization of elastic fibers in some tissues. The most common problems arise in the skin and eyes, and later in blood vessels in the form of premature atherosclerosis. PXE is caused by autosomal recessive mutations in the ABCC6 gene on the short arm of chromosome 16 (16p13.1).

Chapter 7. Clinical Assessment of Asthma and COPD

Asthma	Asthma is characterized by a predisposition to chronic inflammation of the lungs in which the airways (bronchi) are reversibly narrowed. Asthma affects 7% of the population of the United States, 6.5% of British people and a total of 300 million worldwide. During Asthma attacks (exacerbations of Asthma), the smooth muscle cells in the bronchi constrict, the airways become inflamed and swollen, and breathing becomes difficult.
Chronic obstructive pulmonary disease	Chronic obstructive pulmonary disease refers to chronic bronchitis and emphysema, a pair of two commonly co-existing diseases of the lungs in which the airways become narrowed. This leads to a limitation of the flow of air to and from the lungs causing shortness of breath. In contrast to asthma, the limitation of airflow is poorly reversible and usually gets progressively worse over time.
Defensins	Defensins are small cysteine-rich cationic proteins found in both vertebrates and invertebrates. They are active against bacteria, fungi and many enveloped and nonenveloped viruses. They consist of 18-45 amino acids including six (in vertebrates) to 8 conserved cysteine residues.
Dendritic cell	Dendritic cells are immune cells that form part of the mammalian immune system. Their main function is to process antigen material and present it on the surface to other cells of the immune system, thus functioning as antigen-presenting cells. They act as messengers between the innate and adaptive immunity. Dendritic cells are present in small quantities in tissues that are in contact with the external environment, mainly the skin (where there is a specialized Dendritic cell type called Langerhans cells) and the inner lining of the nose, lungs, stomach and intestines. They can also be found in an immature state in the blood.
Diagnosis	In medicine, diagnosis (plural, diagnoses) is the process of identifying a medical condition or disease by its signs, symptoms, and from the results of various diagnostic procedures. The conclusion reached through this process is called a diagnosis. The term \`diagnostic criteria\` designates the combination of signs, symptoms, and test results that allows the health care practitioner to ascertain the diagnosis of the respective disease.
Artery	The arterial system is the higher-pressure portion of the circulatory system. Arterial pressure varies between the peak pressure during heart contraction, called the systolic pressure, and the minimum, or diastolic pressure between contractions, when the heart expands and refills. This pressure variation within the Artery produces the pulse which is observable in any Artery, and reflects heart activity.

Coronary artery disease	(Coronary artery disease or atherosclerotic heart disease) is the end result of the accumulation of atheromatous plaques within the walls of the coronary arteries that supply the myocardium (the muscle of the heart) with oxygen and nutrients. It is sometimes also called coronary heart disease (CHD), although Coronary artery disease is the most common cause of CHD, it is not the only one. Coronary artery disease is the leading cause of death worldwide.
Differential diagnosis	A Differential diagnosis is a systematic method used to identify unknowns. This method, essentially a process of elimination, is used by taxonomists to identify living organisms, and by physicians, physician assistants, and other trained medical professionals to diagnose the specific disease in a patient. Not all medical diagnoses are differential ones: some diagnoses merely name a set of signs and symptoms that may have more than one possible cause, and some diagnoses are based on intuition or estimations of likelihood.
Duffy antigen	The Duffy antigen is a protein located on the surface of red blood cells and is named after the patient in which it was discovered. In humans, this protein is encoded by the Duffy antigenRC gene. The protein encoded by this gene is a glycosylated membrane protein and a non-specific receptor for several chemokines.
Dyspnea	Dyspnea , also called shortness of breath (SOB) or air hunger, is a debilitating symptom that is the experience of unpleasant or uncomfortable respiratory sensations. It is a common symptom of numerous medical disorders, particularly those involving the cardiovascular and respiratory systems; Dyspnea on exertion is the most common presenting complaint for people with respiratory impairment. Dyspnea has been more specifically defined by the American Thoracic Society as the `subjective experience of breathing discomfort that consists of qualitatively distinct sensations that vary in intensity.

Bronchodilator	A Bronchodilator is a substance that dilates the bronchi and bronchioles, decreasing airway resistance and thereby facilitating airflow. Bronchodilators may be endogenous (originating naturally within the body), or they may be medications administered for the treatment of breathing difficulties. They are most useful in obstructive lung diseases, of which asthma and chronic obstructive pulmonary disease are the most common conditions.
Factor XII	Hageman factor is a plasma protein , an enzyme (EC 3.4.21.38) of the serine protease (or serine endopeptidase) class. In humans, Factor XII is encoded by the F12 gene. It is part of the coagulation cascade and activates factor XI and prekallikrein.
Growth factor	A Growth factor is a naturally occurring substance capable of stimulating cellular growth, proliferation and cellular differentiation. Usually it is a protein or a steroid hormone. Growth factors are important for regulating a variety of cellular processes.
Lung	The Lung or pulmonary system is the essential respiration organ in all air-breathing animals, including most tetrapods, a few fish and a few snails. In mammals and the more complex life forms, the two Lungs are located in the chest on either side of the heart. Their principal function is to transport oxygen from the atmosphere into the bloodstream, and to release carbon dioxide from the bloodstream into the atmosphere.
Protein	Proteins are organic compounds made of amino acids arranged in a linear chain and folded into a globular form. The amino acids in a polymer chain are joined together by the peptide bonds between the carboxyl and amino groups of adjacent amino acid residues. The sequence of amino acids in a protein is defined by the sequence of a gene, which is encoded in the genetic code.
Spirometry	Spirometry (meaning the measuring of breath) is the most common of the Pulmonary Function Tests (PFTs), measuring lung function, specifically the measurement of the amount (volume) and/or speed (flow) of air that can be inhaled and exhaled. Spirometry is an important tool used for generating pneumotachographs which are helpful in assessing conditions such as asthma, pulmonary fibrosis, cystic fibrosis, and COPD. Device for Spirometry. The patient places his or her lips around the blue mouthpiece.
Surfactant	Surfactants are wetting agents that lower the surface tension of a liquid, allowing easier spreading, and lower the interfacial tension between two liquids.

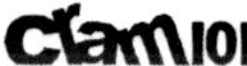

	The term Surfactant is a blend of surface active agent. Surfactants are usually organic compounds that are amphiphilic, meaning they contain both hydrophobic groups (their `tails`) and hydrophilic groups (their `heads`).
Atherosclerosis	Atherosclerosis is a condition in which an artery wall thickens as the result of a build-up of fatty materials such as cholesterol. It is a syndrome affecting arterial blood vessels, a chronic inflammatory response in the walls of arteries, in large part due to the accumulation of macrophage white blood cells and promoted by low-density lipoproteins (plasma proteins that carry cholesterol and triglycerides) without adequate removal of fats and cholesterol from the macrophages by functional high density lipoproteins (HDL), . It is commonly referred to as a hardening or furring of the arteries.
Acute respiratory distress syndrome	Acute respiratory distress syndrome , also known as respiratory distress syndrome (RDS) or adult respiratory distress syndrome (in contrast with IRDS) is a serious reaction to various forms of injuries to the lung. Acute respiratory distress syndrome is a severe lung disease caused by a variety of direct and indirect issues. It is characterized by inflammation of the lung parenchyma leading to impaired gas exchange with concomitant systemic release of inflammatory mediators causing inflammation, hypoxemia and frequently resulting in multiple organ failure.
Allergen	An Allergen is a nonparasitic antigen capable of stimulating a type-I hypersensitivity reaction in atopic individuals. Most humans mount significant Immunoglobulin E responses only as a defense against parasitic infections. However, some individuals mount an IgE response against common environmental antigens.
Arterial blood	In the circulatory system, Arterial Blood is the oxygenated blood in the lungs, found in the left chambers of the heart and in the arteries. It is bright red in color, venous blood is dark red in color (but looks purple through the opaque skin). It is the contralateral term to Venous blood.
Arterial blood gas	An Arterial blood gas is a blood test that is performed using blood from an artery. It involves puncturing an artery with a thin needle and syringe and drawing a small volume of blood. The most common puncture site is the radial artery at the wrist, but sometimes the femoral artery in the groin or other sites are used.
Corticosteroid	Corticosteroids are a class of steroid hormones that are produced in the adrenal cortex. Corticosteroids are involved in a wide range of physiologic systems such as stress response, immune response and regulation of inflammation, carbohydrate metabolism, protein catabolism, blood electrolyte levels, and behavior.

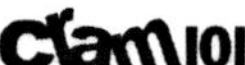

· Glucocorticoids such as cortisol control carbohydrate, fat and protein metabolism and are anti-inflammatory by preventing phospholipid release, decreasing eosinophil action and a number of other mechanisms.

· Mineralocorticoids such as aldosterone control electrolyte and water levels, mainly by promoting sodium retention in the kidney.

Some common natural hormones are corticosterone ($C_{21}H_{30}O_4$), cortisone ($C_{21}H_{28}O_5$, 17-hydroxy-11-dehydrocorticosterone) and aldosterone.

Monitoring

To monitor or Monitoring generally means to be aware of the state of a system. Below are specific examples:

· to observe a situation for any changes which may occur over time, using a monitor or measuring device of some sort:

· Baby monitor, medical monitor, Heart rate monitor

· BioMonitoring

· Cure Monitoring for composite materials manufacturing

· Deformation Monitoring

· Election Monitoring

· Mining Monitoring

· Natural hazard Monitoring

· Network Monitoring

· Structural Monitoring

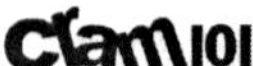

· Website Monitoring

· Futures Monitoring, Media Monitoring service

· to observe the behaviour or communications of individuals or groups

· Monitoring competence at a task.

· Clinical Monitoring for new medical drugs
Monitoring Integration Platform

· Indiktor - Monitoring Integration Platform

·

Bacterial infection

Pathogenic bacteria are bacteria that cause bacterial infection

Although the vast majority of bacteria are harmless or beneficial, quite a few bacteria are pathogenic.

Inflammation

Inflammation is the complex biological response of vascular tissues to harmful stimuli, such as pathogens, damaged cells, or irritants. Inflammation is a protective attempt by the organism to remove the injurious stimuli as well as initiate the healing process for the tissue. Inflammation is not a synonym for infection.

Disease

A disease or medical condition is an abnormal condition of an organism that impairs bodily functions, associated with specific symptoms and signs. It may be caused by external factors, such as invading organisms, or it may be caused by internal dysfunctions, such as autoimmune diseases.
In human beings, `disease` is often used more broadly to refer to any condition that causes pain, dysfunction, distress, social problems, and/or death to the person afflicted, or similar problems for those in contact with the person.

Obstructive Lung Disease	Obstructive lung disease is a category of respiratory disease characterized by airway obstruction. MeSH includes the following in this category: · Asthma · Bronchitis · Chronic obstructive pulmonary disease Cystic fibrosis is sometimes also included in this category. FEV1/FVC ratio is usually decreased.
Bone	Bones are rigid organs that form part of the endoskeleton of vertebrates. They function to move, support, and protect the various organs of the body, produce red and white blood cells and store minerals. bone tissue is a type of dense connective tissue.
Metabolism	Metabolism is the set of chemical reactions that happen in living organisms to maintain life. These processes allow organisms to grow and reproduce, maintain their structures, and respond to their environments. Metabolism is usually divided into two categories.
Cancer	Cancer is a genetic disorder in which the normal control of cell growth is lost. Cancer genetics is now one of the fastest expanding medical specialties. At the molecular level, Cancer is caused by mutation(s) in DNA, which result in aberrant cell proliferation.
Heart	The heart is a myogenic muscular organ found in all animals with a circulatory system (including all vertebrates), that is responsible for pumping blood throughout the blood vessels by repeated, rhythmic contractions. The term cardiac (as in cardiology) means "related to the heart" and comes from the Greek καρδι?, kardia, for "heart". The vertebrate heart is composed of cardiac muscle, which is an involuntary striated muscle tissue found only in this organ, and connective tissue.

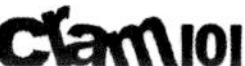

Heart failure	Heart failure is generally defined as inability of the heart to supply sufficient blood flow to meet the body's needs. It has various diagnostic criteria, and the term heart failure is often incorrectly used to describe other cardiac-related illnesses, such as myocardial infarction (heart attack) or cardiac arrest. Common causes of heart failure include myocardial infarction (heart attacks) and other forms of ischemic heart disease, hypertension, valvular heart disease, and cardiomyopathy.
Hypertension	Hypertension is a chronic medical condition in which the blood pressure is elevated. It is also referred to as high blood pressure or shortened to HT, HTN or HPN. The word `Hypertension`, by itself, normally refers to systemic, arterial Hypertension. Hypertension can be classified as either essential (primary) or secondary.
Exhaled nitric oxide	In medicine, Exhaled nitric oxide (eNO) can be measured in a breath test for asthma or other conditions characterized by airway inflammation. Nitric oxide (NO) is a gaseous molecule produced by certain cell types in an inflammatory response. The fraction of exhaled NO (FE_{NO})is a promising biomarker for the diagnosis, follow-up and as a guide to therapy in adults and children with asthma.
Cell type	A Cell type is a distinct morphological or functional form of cell. When a cell switches state from one Cell type to another, it undergoes cellular differentiation. A complete list of distinct Cell types in the adult human body may include about 210 distinct types.
Bronchiectasis	Bronchiectasis is a disease that causes localized, irreversible dilation of part of the bronchial tree. It is classified as an obstructive lung disease, along with bronchitis and cystic fibrosis. Involved bronchi are dilated, inflamed, and easily collapsible, resulting in airflow obstruction and impaired clearance of secretions.
Bronchitis	Bronchitis is inflammation of the mucous membranes of the bronchi, the airways that carry airflow from the trachea into the lungs. Bronchitis can be classified into two categories, acute and chronic, each of which has unique etiologies, pathologies, and therapies. Acute Bronchitis is characterized by the development of a cough, with or without the production of sputum, mucus that is expectorated (coughed up) from the respiratory tract.

Chapter 7. Clinical Assessment of Asthma and COPD

Allergic rhinitis	Allergic rhinitis, pollenosis or hay fever is an allergic inflammation of the nasal airways. It occurs when an allergen such as pollen or dust is inhaled by an individual with a sensitized immune system, and triggers antibody production. The specific antibody is immunoglobulin E (IgE) which binds to mast cells and basophils containing histamine.
Bronchoscopy	Bronchoscopy is a technique of visualizing the inside of the airways for diagnostic and therapeutic purposes. An instrument (bronchoscope) is inserted into the airways, usually through the nose or mouth, or occasionally through a tracheostomy. This allows the practitioner to examine the patient's airways for abnormalities such as foreign bodies, bleeding, tumors, or inflammation.
Cystic fibrosis	Cystic fibrosis (also known as Cystic fibrosis, mucovoidosis,) is a genetic disorder known to be an inherited disease of the secretory glands, including the glands that make mucus and sweat. The hallmarks of Cystic fibrosis are salty tasting skin, normal appetite but poor growth and poor weight gain, excess mucus production, frequent chest infections and coughing/shortness of breath. Males can be infertile due to the condition Congenital absence of the vas deferens.
Dyskinesia	Dyskinesia is a movement disorder which consists of effects including diminished voluntary movements and the presence of involuntary movements, similar to tics or chorea. Dyskinesia is a symptom of several medical disorders and is distinguished by the underlying cause. When a Dyskinesia presents after treatment with an antipsychotic drug such as haloperidol (Haldol), it is known as tardive Dyskinesia, and is commonly seen in the face and mouth in the form of `tongue rolling`.
Fibroblast	A Fibroblast is a type of cell that synthesizes the extracellular matrix and collagen, the structural framework (stroma) for animal tissues, and plays a critical role in wound healing. Fibroblasts are the most common cells of connective tissue in animals. Fibroblasts and fibrocytes are two states of the same cells, the former being the activated state, the latter the less active state, concerned with maintenance.
Leukocytes	White blood cells are cells of the immune system defending the body against both infectious disease and foreign materials. Five different and diverse types of Leukocytes exist, but they are all produced and derived from a multipotent cell in the bone marrow known as a hematopoietic stem cell. Leukocytes are found throughout the body, including the blood and lymphatic system.

Neuroendocrine

Neuroendocrine [IPA nÊŠÉ™roÊŠËˆÉ›ndÉ™krÉªn] cells are cells that release a hormone into the circulating blood in response to a neural stimulus. These hormones may be amines, neuropeptides, or specialized amino acids. They package the hormones in vesicles and send these packages via long processes to blood vessels.

Sarcoidosis

Sarcoidosis is a systemic disease of unknown aetiology that results in the formation of non-caseating granulomas in multiple organs. The prevalence is higher among blacks than whites by a ratio of 20:1. Usually the disease is localized to the chest, but urogenital involvement is found in 0.2% of clinically diagnosed cases and 5% of those diagnosed at necropsy.

Tuberculosis

Tuberculosis or TB (short for Tubercle Bacillus) is a common and often deadly infectious disease caused by mycobacteria, usually Mycobacterium Tuberculosis in humans. Tuberculosis usually attacks the lungs but can also affect other parts of the body. It is spread through the air, when people who have the disease cough, sneeze, or spit.

Viral

The term Viral is used to describe anything related to viruses.

Viral may also mean:

. .

Serum

In blood, the serum is the component that is neither a blood cell nor a clotting factor; it is the blood plasma with the fibrinogens removed. serum includes all proteins not used in blood clotting and all the electrolytes, antibodies, antigens, hormones, and any exogenous substances (e.g., drugs and microorganisms).
The study of serum is serology.

Emphysema

Emphysema is a lung disease, characterized by an abnormal, permanent enlargement of air spaces distal to the terminal bronchioles. The disease is coupled with the destruction of walls, but without obvious fibrosis. It is often caused by exposure to toxic chemicals, including long-term exposure to tobacco smoke.

Surgery	Surgery is the branch of medicine that deals with the physical manipulation of a bodily structure to diagnose, prevent, a 16th century French surgeon, stated that there were five reasons to perform Surgery: `To eliminate that which is superfluous, restore that which has been dislocated, separate that which has been united, join that which has been divided and repair the defects of nature.` Since human beings first learned to make and handle tools, they have employed their talents to develop surgical techniques, each time more sophisticated than the last; however, up until the industrial revolution, surgeons were incapable of overcoming the three principal obstacles which had plagued the medical profession from its infancy -- bleeding, pain and infection. Advances in these fields have transformed Surgery from a risky `art` into a scientific discipline capable of treating many diseases and conditions.
Volume	The Volume of any solid, liquid, gas, plasma, or vacuum is how much three-dimensional space it occupies, often quantified numerically. One-dimensional figures (such as lines) and two-dimensional shapes (such as squares) are assigned zero Volume in the three-dimensional space. Volume is commonly presented in units such as cubic meters, cubic centimeters, liters, or milliliters.
Cardiovascular disease	Heart disease or cardiovascular diseases is the class of diseases that involve the heart or blood vessels (arteries and veins). While the term technically refers to any disease that affects the cardiovascular system (as used in MeSH C14), it is usually used to refer to those related to atherosclerosis (arterial disease). These conditions usually have similar causes, mechanisms, and treatments.
Ejection fraction	In cardiovascular physiology, ejection fraction is the fraction of blood pumped out of the right and left ventricles with each heart beat. The term ejection fraction applies to both the right and left ventricles; one can speak equally of the left ventricular ejection fraction and the right ventricular ejection fraction. RVEF and LVEF may vary widely from one another incumbent upon physiologic state.
Salbutamol	Salbutamol (INN) or albuterol (USAN) is a short-acting β_2-adrenergic receptor agonist used for the relief of bronchospasm in conditions such as asthma and chronic obstructive pulmonary disease. It is marketed by GlaxoSmithKline as Ventolin, Aerolin or Ventorlin depending on the market; by Cipla as Asthalin; by Schering-Plough as Proventil and by Teva as ProAir. Generic names are currently not available in the U.S. because of a federal ban on the use of CFCs.
Subclinical infection	A Subclinical infection is the asymptomatic (without apparent sign) carrying of an (infection) by an individual of an agent (microbe, intestinal parasite,) that usually is a pathogen causing illness, at least in some individuals. Many pathogens spread by being silently carried in this way by some of their host population. Such infections occur both in humans and nonhuman animals.

Metabolic syndrome	Metabolic syndrome is a combination of medical disorders that increase the risk of developing cardiovascular disease and diabetes. It affects one in five people, and prevalence increases with age. Some studies estimate the prevalence in the USA to be up to 25% of the population.
Omalizumab	Omalizumab (Xolair, Genentech / Novartis) is a humanized antibody drug approved for patients with moderate-to-severe or severe allergic asthma, which is caused by hypersensitivity reactions to certain harmless environmental substances. Omalizumab`s cost is high ($10,000 to $30,000 per year), as compared to other drugs used for asthma, and hence Omalizumab is mainly prescribed for patients with severe, persistent asthma, which cannot be controlled even with high doses of corticosteroids. Like other protein and antibody drugs, Omalizumab causes anaphylaxis (a life-threatening systemic allergic reaction) in 1 to 2 patients per 1,000.
Osteoporosis	Osteoporosis is a disease of bone that leads to an increased risk of fracture. In osteoporosis the bone mineral density (BMD) is reduced, bone microarchitecture is disrupted, and the amount and variety of proteins in bone is altered. osteoporosis is defined by the World Health Organization (WHO) in women as a bone mineral density 2.5 standard deviations below peak bone mass (20-year-old healthy female average) as measured by DXA; the term 'established osteoporosis' includes the presence of a fragility fracture.
Colitis	Colitis is a chronic digestive disease characterized by inflammation of the colon. Colitis is one of a group of conditions which are inflammatory and auto-immune, affecting the tissue that lines the gastrointestinal system (the large and small intestine). It is classed as an inflammatory bowel disease (IBD), not to be confused with irritable bowel syndrome (IBS).
Ulcerative colitis	Ulcerative colitis (Colitis ulcerosa, Ulcerative colitis) is a form of inflammatory bowel disease (IBD). Ulcerative colitis is a form of colitis, a disease of the intestine, specifically the large intestine or colon, that includes characteristic ulcers, or open sores, in the colon. The main symptom of active disease is usually constant diarrhea mixed with blood, of gradual onset.
Usual interstitial pneumonia	Usual interstitial pneumonia, commonly abbreviated Usual interstitial pneumonia, is the name of a histopathological pattern seen in diffuse lung diseases, i.e. interstitial lung diseases. It is classified as an idiopathic interstitial pneumonia, and may be idiopathic, i.e. the cause is unknown, or due to a known cause, e.g. asbestos exposure. The hallmarks of Usual interstitial pneumonia are interstitial inflammation, i.e. inflammation of the alveolar walls, and fibrosis (scarring).
Vascular endothelial growth factor	Vascular endothelial growth factor is a signal protein produced by cells that stimulates the growth of new blood vessels. It is part of the system that restores the oxygen supply to tissues when blood circulation is inadequate.

	Vascular endothelial growth factor's normal function is to create new blood vessels during embryonic development, new blood vessels after injury, muscle following exercise, and new vessels (collateral circulation) to bypass blocked vessels.
Intestine	In anatomy, the intestine is the segment of the alimentary canal extending from the stomach to the anus and, in humans and other mammals, consists of two segments, the small intestine and the large intestine. In humans, the small intestine is further subdivided into the duodenum, jejunum and ileum while the large intestine is subdivided into the cecum and colon. The structure and function can be described both as gross anatomy and at a microscopic level.
Pelvic inflammatory disease	Pelvic inflammatory disease (or disorder) is a generic term for inflammation of the female uterus, fallopian tubes, and/or ovaries as it progresses to scar formation with adhesions to nearby tissues and organs. This may lead to tissue necrosis and sometimes abscess formation whereby pus can be released into the peritoneum. Pelvic inflammatory disease is often associated with sexually transmitted infections, as it is a common result of such infections.
Inflammatory bowel disease	In medicine, Inflammatory bowel disease is a group of inflammatory conditions of the colon and small intestine. The major types of Inflammatory bowel disease are Crohn`s disease and ulcerative colitis.. The main forms of Inflammatory bowel disease are Crohn`s disease and ulcerative colitis (UC).
Panic disorder	Panic disorder is an anxiety disorder characterized by recurring severe panic attacks. It may also include significant behavioral change lasting at least a month and of ongoing worry about the implications or concern about having other attacks. The latter are called anticipatory attacks (DSM-IVR).

Chapter 8. Therapies for Asthma and COPD

Asthma	Asthma is characterized by a predisposition to chronic inflammation of the lungs in which the airways (bronchi) are reversibly narrowed. Asthma affects 7% of the population of the United States, 6.5% of British people and a total of 300 million worldwide. During Asthma attacks (exacerbations of Asthma), the smooth muscle cells in the bronchi constrict, the airways become inflamed and swollen, and breathing becomes difficult.
Chronic obstructive pulmonary disease	Chronic obstructive pulmonary disease refers to chronic bronchitis and emphysema, a pair of two commonly co-existing diseases of the lungs in which the airways become narrowed. This leads to a limitation of the flow of air to and from the lungs causing shortness of breath. In contrast to asthma, the limitation of airflow is poorly reversible and usually gets progressively worse over time.
Heart	The heart is a myogenic muscular organ found in all animals with a circulatory system (including all vertebrates), that is responsible for pumping blood throughout the blood vessels by repeated, rhythmic contractions. The term cardiac (as in cardiology) means "related to the heart" and comes from the Greek καρδι?, kardia, for "heart". The vertebrate heart is composed of cardiac muscle, which is an involuntary striated muscle tissue found only in this organ, and connective tissue.
Heart disease	Heart disease is an umbrella term for a variety of diseases affecting the heart. As of 2007, it is the leading cause of death in the United States, England, Canada and Wales, accounting for 25.4% of the total deaths in the United States. Types Coronary heart disease Coronary heart disease refers to the failure of the coronary circulation to supply adequate circulation to cardiac muscle and surrounding tissue.

Cholesterol	Cholesterol is a lipidic, waxy steroid found in the cell membranes and transported in the blood plasma of all animals. It is an essential component of mammalian cell membranes where it is required to establish proper membrane permeability and fluidity. In addition, Cholesterol is an important precursor molecule for the biosynthesis of bile acids, steroid hormones, and several fat soluble vitamins.
Hypercholesterolemia	Hypercholesterolemia (literally: high blood cholesterol) is the presence of high levels of cholesterol in the blood. It is not a disease but a metabolic derangement that can be secondary to many diseases and can contribute to many forms of disease, most notably cardiovascular disease. It is closely related to the terms \`hyperlipidemia\` (elevated levels of lipids) and \`hyperlipoproteinemia\` (elevated levels of lipoproteins).
Hypertension	Hypertension is a chronic medical condition in which the blood pressure is elevated. It is also referred to as high blood pressure or shortened to HT, HTN or HPN. The word \`Hypertension\`, by itself, normally refers to systemic, arterial Hypertension. Hypertension can be classified as either essential (primary) or secondary.
Atherosclerosis	Atherosclerosis is a condition in which an artery wall thickens as the result of a build-up of fatty materials such as cholesterol. It is a syndrome affecting arterial blood vessels, a chronic inflammatory response in the walls of arteries, in large part due to the accumulation of macrophage white blood cells and promoted by low-density lipoproteins (plasma proteins that carry cholesterol and triglycerides) without adequate removal of fats and cholesterol from the macrophages by functional high density lipoproteins (HDL), . It is commonly referred to as a hardening or furring of the arteries.
Acute respiratory distress syndrome	Acute respiratory distress syndrome , also known as respiratory distress syndrome (RDS) or adult respiratory distress syndrome (in contrast with IRDS) is a serious reaction to various forms of injuries to the lung. Acute respiratory distress syndrome is a severe lung disease caused by a variety of direct and indirect issues. It is characterized by inflammation of the lung parenchyma leading to impaired gas exchange with concomitant systemic release of inflammatory mediators causing inflammation, hypoxemia and frequently resulting in multiple organ failure.
Arterial stiffness	Arteries stiffen as a consequence of age and atherosclerosis. The two leading causes of death in the developed world, myocardial infarction and stroke, are both a direct consequence of atherosclerosis. Increased Arterial stiffness is associated with an increased risk of cardiovascular events.

Atrial fibrillation	Atrial fibrillation is the most common cardiac arrhythmia (abnormal heart rhythm), and involves the two upper chambers (atria) of the heart. Its name comes from the fibrillating (i.e., quivering) of the heart muscles of the atria, instead of a coordinated contraction. It can often be identified by taking a pulse and observing that the heartbeats do not occur at regular intervals.
Cancer	Cancer is a genetic disorder in which the normal control of cell growth is lost. Cancer genetics is now one of the fastest expanding medical specialties. At the molecular level, Cancer is caused by mutation(s) in DNA, which result in aberrant cell proliferation.
Emphysema	Emphysema is a lung disease, characterized by an abnormal, permanent enlargement of air spaces distal to the terminal bronchioles. The disease is coupled with the destruction of walls, but without obvious fibrosis. It is often caused by exposure to toxic chemicals, including long-term exposure to tobacco smoke.
Lung	The Lung or pulmonary system is the essential respiration organ in all air-breathing animals, including most tetrapods, a few fish and a few snails. In mammals and the more complex life forms, the two Lungs are located in the chest on either side of the heart. Their principal function is to transport oxygen from the atmosphere into the bloodstream, and to release carbon dioxide from the bloodstream into the atmosphere.
Platelet	Platelets, or thrombocytes , are small, irregularly-shaped anuclear cells , 2-3 Âµm in diameter, which are derived from fragmentation of precursor megakaryocytes. The average lifespan of a Platelet is between 8 and 12 days. Platelets play a fundamental role in hemostasis and are a natural source of growth factors.
Ventricular fibrillation	Ventricular fibrillation is a condition in which there is uncoordinated contraction of the cardiac muscle of the ventricles in the heart, making them quiver rather than contract properly. While there is activity, it is undetectable by palpation (feeling) at major pulse points of the carotid and femoral arteries especially by the lay person. Such an arrhythmia is only confirmed by electrocardiography.
C-reactive protein	C-reactive protein (CRP) is a protein found in the blood, the levels of which rise in response to inflammation (an acute-phase protein). CRP is synthesized by the liver in response to factors released by fat cells (adipocytes). It is a member of the pentraxin family of proteins.
Duffy antigen	The Duffy antigen is a protein located on the surface of red blood cells and is named after the patient in which it was discovered. In humans, this protein is encoded by the Duffy antigenRC gene.

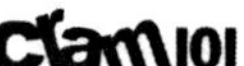

The protein encoded by this gene is a glycosylated membrane protein and a non-specific receptor for several chemokines.

Bronchial hyperresponsiveness

Bronchial hyperresponsiveness (or other combinations with airway or hyperreactivity) is a state characterised by easily triggered bronchospasm (contraction of the bronchioles or small airways).

Bronchial hyperresponsiveness can be assessed with a bronchial challenge test. This most often uses products like metacholine or histamine.

Dyspnea

Dyspnea , also called shortness of breath (SOB) or air hunger, is a debilitating symptom that is the experience of unpleasant or uncomfortable respiratory sensations. It is a common symptom of numerous medical disorders, particularly those involving the cardiovascular and respiratory systems; Dyspnea on exertion is the most common presenting complaint for people with respiratory impairment.

Dyspnea has been more specifically defined by the American Thoracic Society as the `subjective experience of breathing discomfort that consists of qualitatively distinct sensations that vary in intensity.

Inflammation

Inflammation is the complex biological response of vascular tissues to harmful stimuli, such as pathogens, damaged cells, or irritants. Inflammation is a protective attempt by the organism to remove the injurious stimuli as well as initiate the healing process for the tissue. Inflammation is not a synonym for infection.

Angiotensin

Angiotensin, a protein, causes blood vessels to constrict, and drives blood pressure up. It is part of the renin-Angiotensin system, which is a major target for drugs that lower blood pressure. Angiotensin also stimulates the release of aldosterone from the adrenal cortex.

Artery

The arterial system is the higher-pressure portion of the circulatory system. Arterial pressure varies between the peak pressure during heart contraction, called the systolic pressure, and the minimum, or diastolic pressure between contractions, when the heart expands and refills. This pressure variation within the Artery produces the pulse which is observable in any Artery, and reflects heart activity.

Coronary artery disease	(Coronary artery disease or atherosclerotic heart disease) is the end result of the accumulation of atheromatous plaques within the walls of the coronary arteries that supply the myocardium (the muscle of the heart) with oxygen and nutrients. It is sometimes also called coronary heart disease (CHD), although Coronary artery disease is the most common cause of CHD, it is not the only one. Coronary artery disease is the leading cause of death worldwide.
Multiple inert gas elimination technique	Multiple inert gas elimination technique is a technique used mainly in pneumology, that involves measuring mixed venous, arterial, and mixed expired concentrations of six infused inert gases, shows a shunt, dead space, and the general ventilation versus blood flow (Va/Q). It is a good technique for establishing emphysema or chronic bronchitis.
Allergen	An Allergen is a nonparasitic antigen capable of stimulating a type-I hypersensitivity reaction in atopic individuals. Most humans mount significant Immunoglobulin E responses only as a defense against parasitic infections. However, some individuals mount an IgE response against common environmental antigens.
Colitis	Colitis is a chronic digestive disease characterized by inflammation of the colon. Colitis is one of a group of conditions which are inflammatory and auto-immune, affecting the tissue that lines the gastrointestinal system (the large and small intestine). It is classed as an inflammatory bowel disease (IBD), not to be confused with irritable bowel syndrome (IBS).
Defensins	Defensins are small cysteine-rich cationic proteins found in both vertebrates and invertebrates. They are active against bacteria, fungi and many enveloped and nonenveloped viruses. They consist of 18-45 amino acids including six (in vertebrates) to 8 conserved cysteine residues.
Dendritic cell	Dendritic cells are immune cells that form part of the mammalian immune system. Their main function is to process antigen material and present it on the surface to other cells of the immune system, thus functioning as antigen-presenting cells. They act as messengers between the innate and adaptive immunity.

	Dendritic cells are present in small quantities in tissues that are in contact with the external environment, mainly the skin (where there is a specialized Dendritic cell type called Langerhans cells) and the inner lining of the nose, lungs, stomach and intestines. They can also be found in an immature state in the blood.
Factor XII	Hageman factor is a plasma protein , an enzyme (EC 3.4.21.38) of the serine protease (or serine endopeptidase) class. In humans, Factor XII is encoded by the F12 gene. It is part of the coagulation cascade and activates factor XI and prekallikrein.
Growth factor	A Growth factor is a naturally occurring substance capable of stimulating cellular growth, proliferation and cellular differentiation. Usually it is a protein or a steroid hormone. Growth factors are important for regulating a variety of cellular processes.
Ulcerative colitis	Ulcerative colitis (Colitis ulcerosa, Ulcerative colitis) is a form of inflammatory bowel disease (IBD). Ulcerative colitis is a form of colitis, a disease of the intestine, specifically the large intestine or colon, that includes characteristic ulcers, or open sores, in the colon. The main symptom of active disease is usually constant diarrhea mixed with blood, of gradual onset.
Usual interstitial pneumonia	Usual interstitial pneumonia, commonly abbreviated Usual interstitial pneumonia, is the name of a histopathological pattern seen in diffuse lung diseases, i.e. interstitial lung diseases. It is classified as an idiopathic interstitial pneumonia, and may be idiopathic, i.e. the cause is unknown, or due to a known cause, e.g. asbestos exposure. The hallmarks of Usual interstitial pneumonia are interstitial inflammation, i.e. inflammation of the alveolar walls, and fibrosis (scarring).
Intervention	An intervention is an orchestrated attempt by one, or often many, people (usually family and friends) to get someone to seek professional help with an addiction or some kind of traumatic event or crisis, or other serious problem. The term intervention is most often used when the traumatic event involves addiction to drugs or other items. intervention can also refer to the act of using a technique within a therapy session.
Eczema	Eczema is a disease in a form of dermatitis, or inflammation of the epidermis. The term Eczema is broadly applied to a range of persistent skin conditions. These include dryness and recurring skin rashes that are characterized by one or more of these symptoms: redness, skin edema (swelling), itching and dryness, crusting, flaking, blistering, cracking, oozing, or bleeding.
Primary	In medicine, the reporting of symptoms by a patient may have significant psychological motivators. Psychologists sometimes categorize these motivators into primary or secondary gain.

primary gain is internally good; motivationally.

Epidemic

In epidemiology, an Epidemic occurs when new cases of a certain disease, in a given human population, and during a given period, substantially exceed what is `expected,` based on recent experience . (An epizootic is the analogous circumstance within an animal population). In recent usages, the disease is not required to be communicable; examples include cancer or heart disease.

Necrosis

Necrosis is the premature death of cells and living tissue. Necrosis is caused by factors external to the cell or tissue, such as infection, toxins, or trauma. This is in contrast to apoptosis, which is a naturally occurring cause of cellular death.

Smoking cessation

Smoking cessation (or quitting smoking) is the action leading towards the discontinuation of the consumption of a smoked substance, mainly tobacco, but it may encompass cannabis and other substances as well.
Smoking certain substances can be addictive. This encompasses both psychological and biological addiction.

Gingiva

The Gingiva consists of the mucosal tissue that lies over the alveolar bone.

Gingiva are part of the soft tissue lining of the mouth. They surround the teeth and provide a seal around them.

Insomnia

Insomnia is a symptom of any of several sleep disorders, characterized by persistent difficulty falling asleep or staying asleep despite the opportunity. Insomnia is a symptom, not a stand-alone diagnosis or a disease. By definition, Insomnia is `difficulty initiating or maintaining sleep, or both` and it may be due to inadequate quality or quantity of sleep.

Norepinephrine

Norepinephrine or noradrenaline (BAN) is a catecholamine with multiple roles including as a hormone and a neurotransmitter.

As a stress hormone, Norepinephrine affects parts of the brain where attention and responding actions are controlled. Along with epinephrine, Norepinephrine also underlies the fight-or-flight response, directly increasing heart rate, triggering the release of glucose from energy stores, and increasing blood flow to skeletal muscle.

Paracetamol	Paracetamol or acetaminophen) is a widely used over-the-counter analgesic (pain reliever) and antipyretic (fever reducer). However, its effectiveness alone as an antipyretic has been questioned. It is commonly used for the relief of headaches, and other minor aches and pains, and is a major ingredient in numerous cold and flu remedies.
Selective serotonin reuptake inhibitors	Selective serotonin reuptake inhibitors anxiety disorders, and some personality disorders. They are also typically effective and used in treating premature ejaculation problems as well as some cases of insomnia. SSRIs increase the extracellular level of the neurotransmitter serotonin by inhibiting its reuptake into the presynaptic cell, increasing the level of serotonin available to bind to the postsynaptic receptor.
Vascular endothelial growth factor	Vascular endothelial growth factor is a signal protein produced by cells that stimulates the growth of new blood vessels. It is part of the system that restores the oxygen supply to tissues when blood circulation is inadequate. Vascular endothelial growth factor's normal function is to create new blood vessels during embryonic development, new blood vessels after injury, muscle following exercise, and new vessels (collateral circulation) to bypass blocked vessels.
Adenosine	Adenosine is a nucleoside composed of a molecule of adenine attached to a ribose sugar molecule (ribofuranose) moiety via a β-N_9-glycosidic bond. Adenosine plays an important role in biochemical processes, such as energy transfer--as adenosine triphosphate (ATP) and adenosine diphosphate (ADP)--as well as in signal transduction as cyclic adenosine monophosphate, cAMP. It is also an inhibitory neurotransmitter, believed to play a role in promoting sleep and suppressing arousal, with levels increasing with each hour an organism is awake. Adenosine is often abbreviated Ado.

Chapter 8. Therapies for Asthma and COPD

Ejection fraction

In cardiovascular physiology, ejection fraction is the fraction of blood pumped out of the right and left ventricles with each heart beat. The term ejection fraction applies to both the right and left ventricles; one can speak equally of the left ventricular ejection fraction and the right ventricular ejection fraction. RVEF and LVEF may vary widely from one another incumbent upon physiologic state.

Mechanism of action

In pharmacology, the term Mechanism of action refers to the specific biochemical interaction through which a drug substance produces its pharmacological effect. A Mechanism of action usually includes mention of the specific molecular targets to which the drug binds, such as an enzyme or receptor.

For example, the Mechanism of action of aspirin involves irreversible inhibition of the enzyme cyclooxygenase, which suppresses the production of prostaglandins and thromboxanes, thereby reducing pain and inflammation.

Salbutamol

Salbutamol (INN) or albuterol (USAN) is a short-acting β_2-adrenergic receptor agonist used for the relief of bronchospasm in conditions such as asthma and chronic obstructive pulmonary disease. It is marketed by GlaxoSmithKline as Ventolin, Aerolin or Ventorlin depending on the market; by Cipla as Asthalin; by Schering-Plough as Proventil and by Teva as ProAir. Generic names are currently not available in the U.S. because of a federal ban on the use of CFCs.

Subclinical infection

A Subclinical infection is the asymptomatic (without apparent sign) carrying of an (infection) by an individual of an agent (microbe, intestinal parasite,) that usually is a pathogen causing illness, at least in some individuals. Many pathogens spread by being silently carried in this way by some of their host population. Such infections occur both in humans and nonhuman animals.

Volume

The Volume of any solid, liquid, gas, plasma, or vacuum is how much three-dimensional space it occupies, often quantified numerically. One-dimensional figures (such as lines) and two-dimensional shapes (such as squares) are assigned zero Volume in the three-dimensional space. Volume is commonly presented in units such as cubic meters, cubic centimeters, liters, or milliliters.

Salmeterol

Salmeterol is a long-acting beta2-adrenergic receptor agonist drug that is currently prescribed for the treatment of asthma and chronic obstructive pulmonary disease (COPD). It is currently available as a metered-dose inhaler (MDI) or a proprietary `disk-styled` inhaler that releases a powdered form of the drug.

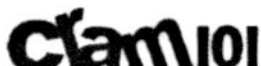

It is a long acting beta-adrenoceptor agonist (LABA), usually only prescribed for severe persistent asthma following previous treatment with a short-acting beta agonist such as salbutamol and is prescribed concurrently with a corticosteroid, such as beclomethasone.

Bronchiectasis

Bronchiectasis is a disease that causes localized, irreversible dilation of part of the bronchial tree. It is classified as an obstructive lung disease, along with bronchitis and cystic fibrosis. Involved bronchi are dilated, inflamed, and easily collapsible, resulting in airflow obstruction and impaired clearance of secretions.

Bronchodilator

A Bronchodilator is a substance that dilates the bronchi and bronchioles, decreasing airway resistance and thereby facilitating airflow. Bronchodilators may be endogenous (originating naturally within the body), or they may be medications administered for the treatment of breathing difficulties. They are most useful in obstructive lung diseases, of which asthma and chronic obstructive pulmonary disease are the most common conditions.

Cystic fibrosis

Cystic fibrosis (also known as Cystic fibrosis, mucovoidosis,) is a genetic disorder known to be an inherited disease of the secretory glands, including the glands that make mucus and sweat. The hallmarks of Cystic fibrosis are salty tasting skin, normal appetite but poor growth and poor weight gain, excess mucus production, frequent chest infections and coughing/shortness of breath. Males can be infertile due to the condition Congenital absence of the vas deferens.

Glucuronide

A Glucuronide is any substance produced by linking glucuronic acid to another substance via a glycosidic bond. The Glucuronides belong to the glycosides.
Glucuronidation, the conversion of chemical compounds to Glucuronides, is a method that animals use to assist in the excretion of toxic substances, drugs or other substances that cannot be used as an energy source.

Fenoterol

Fenoterol is an asthma medication designed to open up the airways to the lungs. It is classed as a beta agonist.
Fenoterol was marketed as `Berotec` by Boehringer-Ingelheim.

Leukocytes

White blood cells are cells of the immune system defending the body against both infectious disease and foreign materials. Five different and diverse types of Leukocytes exist, but they are all produced and derived from a multipotent cell in the bone marrow known as a hematopoietic stem cell. Leukocytes are found throughout the body, including the blood and lymphatic system.

Neuroendocrine	Neuroendocrine [IPA nÊŠÉ™roÊŠË ˆÉ›ndÉ™krÉªn] cells are cells that release a hormone into the circulating blood in response to a neural stimulus. These hormones may be amines, neuropeptides, or specialized amino acids. They package the hormones in vesicles and send these packages via long processes to blood vessels.
Obstructive lung disease	Obstructive lung disease is a category of respiratory disease characterized by airway obstruction. MeSH includes the following in this category: · Asthma · Bronchitis · Chronic obstructive pulmonary disease Cystic fibrosis is sometimes also included in this category. FEV1/FVC ratio is usually decreased.
Atropine	Atropine is a tropane alkaloid extracted from deadly nightshade (Atropa belladonna), jimsonweed (Datura stramonium), mandrake (Mandragora officinarum) and other plants of the family Solanaceae. It is a secondary metabolite of these plants and serves as a drug with a wide variety of effects. It is a competitive antagonist for the muscarinic acetylcholine receptor.
Dose	A dose is a quantity of something (chemical, physical, or biological) that may impact an organism biologically; the greater the quantity, the larger the dose. In nutrition, the term is usually applied to how much of a specific nutrient is in a person's diet or in a particular food, meal, or dietary supplement. In medicine, the term is usually applied to the quantity of a drug or other agent administered for therapeutic purposes.
Inhaler	An Inhaler or puffer is a medical device used for delivering medication into the body via the lungs. It is mainly used in the treatment of asthma and Chronic Obstructive Pulmonary Disease (COPD). To reduce deposition in the mouth and throat, and to reduce the need for precise synchronization of the start of inhalation with actuation of the device, MDIs are sometimes used with a complementary spacer or holding chamber device.

Metered Dose Inhaler	A metered-dose inhaler is a device that delivers a specific amount of medication to the lungs, in the form of a short burst of aerosolized medicine that is inhaled by the patient. It is the most commonly used delivery system for treating asthma, chronic obstructive pulmonary disease (COPD) and other respiratory diseases. The medication in a Metered dose inhaler is most commonly a bronchodilator, corticosteroid or a combination of both for the treatment of asthma and COPD. Other medications less commonly used but also administered by Metered dose inhaler are mast cell stabilizers, such as (cromoglicate or nedocromil).
Anti-inflammatory	Anti-inflammatory refers to the property of a substance or treatment that reduces inflammation. Anti-inflammatory drugs make up about half of analgesics, remedying pain by reducing inflammation as opposed to opioids which affect the brain. Steroids Many steroids, specifically glucocorticoids, reduce inflammation or swelling by binding to cortisol receptors.
Caries	Caries is a progressive destruction of any kind of bone structure, including the skull, ribs and other bones, which is a bacterial disease. A disease that involves Caries is mastoiditis, an inflammation of the mastoid process, in which the bone gets eroded.
Pharmacokinetics	Pharmacokinetics is a branch of pharmacology dedicated to the determination of the fate of substances administered externally to a living organism. In practice, this discipline is applied mainly to drug substances, though in principle it concerns itself with all manner of compounds ingested or otherwise delivered externally to an organism, such as nutrients, metabolites, hormones, toxins, etc. Pharmacokinetics is often studied in conjunction with pharmacodynamics.
Efficacy	Efficacy is the capacity to produce an effect. It has different specific meanings in different fields. In a healthcare context, Efficacy indicates the capacity for beneficial change (or therapeutic effect) of a given intervention.

Budesonide

Budesonide is a glucocorticoid steroid for the treatment of asthma, non-infectious rhinitis (including hay fever and other allergies), and for treatment and prevention of nasal polyposis. Additionally, it is used for Crohn's disease (inflammatory bowel disease). It is marketed by AstraZeneca as a nasal inhalant under the brand name Rhinocort (in Denmark, as Rhinosol), as an oral inhalant under the brand name Pulmicort, and as either an enema or a modified release oral capsule under the brand name Entocort.

Erythromycin

Erythromycin is a macrolide antibiotic that has an antimicrobial spectrum similar to or slightly wider than that of penicillin, and is often used for people who have an allergy to penicillins. For respiratory tract infections, it has better coverage of atypical organisms, including mycoplasma and Legionellosis. It was first marketed by Eli Lilly and Company, and it is today commonly known as EES (Erythromycin ethylsuccinate, an ester prodrug that is commonly administered).

Phosphodiesterase inhibitor

A Phosphodiesterase inhibitor is a drug that blocks one or more of the five subtypes of the enzyme phosphodiesterase (PDE), therefore preventing the inactivation of the intracellular second messengers cyclic adenosine monophosphate (cAMP) and cyclic guanosine monophosphate (cGMP) by the respective PDE subtype(s).

The different forms or subtypes of phosphodiesterase were initially isolated from rat brains by Uzunov and Weiss in 1972 and were soon afterwards shown to be selectively inhibited in the brain and in other tissues by a variety of drugs. The potential for selective Phosphodiesterase inhibitors as therapeutic agents was predicted as early as 1977 by Weiss and Hait.

Clearance

In medicine, the clearance is a measurement of the renal excretion ability. Although clearance may also involve other organs than the kidney, it is almost synonymous with renal clearance or renal plasma clearance. Each substance has a specific clearance that depends on its filtration characteristics.

Corticosteroid

Corticosteroids are a class of steroid hormones that are produced in the adrenal cortex. Corticosteroids are involved in a wide range of physiologic systems such as stress response, immune response and regulation of inflammation, carbohydrate metabolism, protein catabolism, blood electrolyte levels, and behavior.

· Glucocorticoids such as cortisol control carbohydrate, fat and protein metabolism and are anti-inflammatory by preventing phospholipid release, decreasing eosinophil action and a number of other mechanisms.

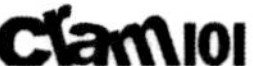

· Mineralocorticoids such as aldosterone control electrolyte and water levels, mainly by promoting sodium retention in the kidney.

Some common natural hormones are corticosterone ($C_{21}H_{30}O_4$), cortisone ($C_{21}H_{28}O_5$, 17-hydroxy-11-dehydrocorticosterone) and aldosterone.

Glucocorticoid

Glucocorticoids are a class of steroid hormones that bind to the Glucocorticoid receptor (GR), which is present in almost every vertebrate animal cell. The name Glucocorticoid derives from their role in the regulation of the metabolism of glucose, their synthesis in the adrenal cortex, and their steroidal structure .

GCs are part of the feedback mechanism in the immune system that turns immune activity (inflammation) down.

Fluticasone

Fluticasone is a synthetic glucocorticoid.
Both the furoate and propionate forms are used as topical anti-inflammatories:

· Fluticasone propionate

· Fluticasone furoate .

Fluticasone propionate

Fluticasone propionate is a synthetic corticosteroid derived from fluticasone used to treat asthma and allergic rhinitis.
GlaxoSmithKline currently markets Fluticasone propionate as Flovent (USA and Canada) and Flixotide (EU) for asthma, and as Flonase (USA and Canada) Flixonase (EU and Brazil) for allergic rhinitis, as well as a combination of fluticasone and salmeterol as Advair (USA and Canada) or Seretide (EU).

It is also available as a cream (marketed as Cutivate or Flutivate) for the treatment of eczema and psoriasis.

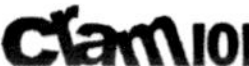

Combination therapy	In contemporary usage, the expression Combination therapy most often refers to the simultaneous administration of two or more medications to treat a single disease, but the expression is also used when other types of therapy are used at the same time. Conditions treated with Combination therapy include tuberculosis, leprosy, cancer, malaria, and HIV/AIDS. Combination therapy may seem costlier than monotherapy in the short term but causes significant savings: lower treatment failure rate, lower case-fatality ratios, slower development of resistance and consequently, less money needed for the development of new drugs.
Disease	A disease or medical condition is an abnormal condition of an organism that impairs bodily functions, associated with specific symptoms and signs. It may be caused by external factors, such as invading organisms, or it may be caused by internal dysfunctions, such as autoimmune diseases. In human beings, `disease` is often used more broadly to refer to any condition that causes pain, dysfunction, distress, social problems, and/or death to the person afflicted, or similar problems for those in contact with the person.
Bone	Bones are rigid organs that form part of the endoskeleton of vertebrates. They function to move, support, and protect the various organs of the body, produce red and white blood cells and store minerals. bone tissue is a type of dense connective tissue.
Metabolism	Metabolism is the set of chemical reactions that happen in living organisms to maintain life. These processes allow organisms to grow and reproduce, maintain their structures, and respond to their environments. Metabolism is usually divided into two categories.
Connective tissue	Connective tissue is a form of fibrous tissue. It is one of the four types of tissue in traditional classifications (the others being epithelial, muscle, and nervous tissue). Collagen is the main protein of Connective tissue in animals and the most abundant protein in mammals, making up about 25% of the total protein content. Fiber types as follows:

· collagenous fibers

· elastic fibers

· Bone Marrow

Various Connective tissue conditions have been identified; these can be both inherited and environmental.

· Marfan syndrome - a genetic disease causing abnormal fibrillin.

· Scurvy - caused by a dietary deficiency in vitamin C, leading to abnormal collagen.

· Ehlers-Danlos syndrome - deficient type III collagen- a genetic disease causing progressive deterioration of collagens, with different EDS types affecting different sites in the body, such as joints, heart valves, organ walls, arterial walls, etc.

· Loeys-Dietz syndrome - a genetic disease related to Marfan syndrome, with an emphasis on vascular deterioration.

· Pseudoxanthoma elasticum - an autosomal recessive hereditary disease, caused by calcification and fragmentation of elastic fibres, affecting the skin, the eyes and the cardiovascular system.

· Systemic lupus erythematosus - a chronic, multisystem, inflammatory disorder of probable autoimmune etiology, occurring predominantly in young women.

· Osteogenesis imperfecta (brittle bone disease) - caused by insufficient production of good quality collagen to produce healthy, strong bones.

· Fibrodysplasia ossificans progressiva - disease of the Connective tissue, caused by a defective gene which turns Connective tissue into bone.

· Spontaneous pneumothorax - collapsed lung, believed to be related to subtle abnormalities in Connective tissue.

· Sarcoma - a neoplastic process originating within Connective tissue.

Pregnancy

Pregnancy is the carrying of one or more offspring, known as a fetus or embryo, inside the uterus of a female. In a Pregnancy, there can be multiple gestations, as in the case of twins or triplets. Human Pregnancy is the most studied of all mammalian pregnancies.

Intramuscular

Intramuscular injection is the injection of a substance directly into a muscle. In medicine, it is one of several alternative methods for the administration of medications . It is used for particular forms of medication that are administered in small amounts.

Omalizumab

Omalizumab (Xolair, Genentech / Novartis) is a humanized antibody drug approved for patients with moderate-to-severe or severe allergic asthma, which is caused by hypersensitivity reactions to certain harmless environmental substances. Omalizumab`s cost is high ($10,000 to $30,000 per year), as compared to other drugs used for asthma, and hence Omalizumab is mainly prescribed for patients with severe, persistent asthma, which cannot be controlled even with high doses of corticosteroids. Like other protein and antibody drugs, Omalizumab causes anaphylaxis (a life-threatening systemic allergic reaction) in 1 to 2 patients per 1,000.

Prednisone

Prednisone is a synthetic corticosteroid drug that is particularly effective as an immunosuppressant, and affects virtually all of the immune system. It is used to treat certain inflammatory diseases and (at higher doses) cancers, but has significant adverse effects. It is usually taken orally but can be delivered by intramuscular injection or intravenous injection.

Rhinovirus

Human Rhinovirus A

Human Rhinovirus B

Human Rhinovirus C

Rhinovirus was a genus of the Picornaviridae family of viruses. It has been now merged into Enteroviruses, a group of Picornaviridae that includes Poliovirus, Coxsackie A virus, and Hepatitis A.

Rhinoviruses are the most common viral infective agents in humans, and a causative agent of the common cold. It is lytic in nature.

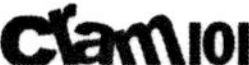

Icatibant	Icatibant (trade name Firazyr) is a peptidomimetic drug consisting of ten amino acids, which is a selective and specific antagonist of bradykinin B2 receptors. It has been approved by the European Commission for the symptomatic treatment of acute attacks , of hereditary angioedema (HAE) in adults (with C1-esterase-inhibitor deficiency). Bradykinin is a peptide-based hormone that is formed locally in tissues, very often in response to a trauma.
Diagnosis	In medicine, diagnosis (plural, diagnoses) is the process of identifying a medical condition or disease by its signs, symptoms, and from the results of various diagnostic procedures. The conclusion reached through this process is called a diagnosis. The term `diagnostic criteria` designates the combination of signs, symptoms, and test results that allows the health care practitioner to ascertain the diagnosis of the respective disease.
Cephalosporin	The Cephalosporins are a class of β-lactam antibiotics originally derived from Acremonium, which was previously known as 'Cephalosporium'. Together with cephamycins they constitute a subgroup of β-lactam antibiotics called cephems. Cephalosporin compounds were first isolated from cultures of Cephalosporium acremonium from a sewer in Sardinia in 1948 by Italian scientist Giuseppe Brotzu .
Quinolone	The Quinolones also referred to as fluoroQuinolones are a family of synthetic broad-spectrum antibiotics. The term Quinolone(s) refers to potent synthetic chemotherapeutic antibacterials the first generation of which was derived from an attempt to create a synthetic form of chloroquine, which was used to treat malaria during World War II. Hans Andersag discovered chloroquine in 1934, at Bayer I.G. Farbenindustrie A.G. laboratories in Eberfeld, Germany. The first generation of the Quinolones begins with the introduction of nalidixic acid in 1962 for treatment of urinary tract infections in humans.
Gas exchange	Gas exchange takes place at a respiratory surface--a boundary between the external environment and the interior of the organism. For unicellular organisms the respiratory surface is governed by Fick`s law, which determines that respiratory surfaces must have: · a large surface area · a thin permeable surface

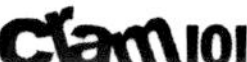

· a moist exchange surface.

Many also have a mechanism to maximise the diffusion gradient by replenishing the source and/or sink.

Control of respiration is due to rhythmical breathing generated by the phrenic nerve in order to stimulate contraction and relaxation of the diaphragm during inspiration and expiration.

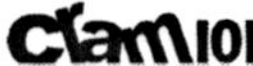

CPSIA information can be obtained
at www.ICGtesting.com
Printed in the USA
LVOW09s1508071216
516245LV00002B/57/P

9 781614 614500